MENTAL HEALTH MAYDAY

A Firefighter's Survival Guide from
Recruit through Retirement

D1620522

GREGG BAGDADE MA, LPC, NCC

For information, contact
MSI Press, LLC
1760-F Airline Hwy #203
Hollister, CA 95023

Copyeditor: Mary Anne Raemisch
Author photo: Tim Olk
Cover design: Peter Streff
Book layout: Opeyemi Ikuborije

LCCN: 2022923638
ISBN: 978-1-957354-22-4

CONTENTS

AUTHOR'S NOTE

Throughout this book, the word *firefighter* is used extensively. Know that this is an all-encompassing term which includes, but is not limited to, *firefighters*, *EMTs* and *paramedics*.

WHY THIS BOOK?

"I am he as you are he as you are me and we are all together."
(Lennon & McCartney, 1967)

When I first got on the Chicago Fire Department, I had trouble coping with the high volume of calls that our ambulance provided for our little slice of the city. I also had issues separating my work-self from my home-self. At my assignment was a paramedic who told me about his routine. He told me that when he got ready to go to a shift in the morning, he put on his uniform like he was Superman. Taking pride in his position as a CFD medic, he donned his work blues and became the superhero he was in his mind. When his shift was done, he would retire to his apartment, take off his uniform and take a shower before putting on his street clothes and readying himself for the rest of the day. This transition was vital for his mental well-being and helped him with the transition from his on-duty life to his off-duty life.

It is these pearls that I wish to bestow on anyone interested in becoming a firefighter. When you begin your career, you are green. You are taught how to force a door, aggressively place water on the seat of a fire, and treat a trauma patient that has fallen six stories to the sidewalk below. As you flourish in your career, you begin to learn the ropes. You make mistakes and make every effort to learn from them so that you become better at your job. When your career is solid, and you have found your place within the chaos, it is your job to hand over your knowledge to the next generation of firefighters. It is our goal, and our responsibility, to make sure that this next generation is better off than we were. But, who teaches us how to control the anger we have due to lack of sleep and quells our frustration when we are unable to resuscitate that eight year old who got into their parent's heroin stash? Who teaches us to not reach for the bottle after we pick up the body parts of a person that has been hit by a train?

Mental health should be in the forefront of every line officer's mind from the moment they report to their assignment throughout their completed tour of duty. Every member of the rank-and-file should be hyperaware of their own mental health as well as that of their peers *and* be capable of knowing what to do if they see one of their comrades in distress. Chief officers are responsible for creating and teaching new content regarding up-to-date mental health material. Just as each day most firehouses are training so as to be prepared for the next time a call comes in and the tones go off, we should be providing daily attention to firefighter mental health.

I was having a discussion with a CFD Fire Captain about the movie *Bringing Out the Dead*, starring Nicolas Cage. The movie showcases a burnt-out paramedic in New York City who simply wants to quit the job. One of the continuous thread plots in the movie is the ghosts he sees of patients that have not survived following his care. They keep coming into his life at the most inopportune times as a reminder of his potential negligence (Scorcese,1999). The Captain had his own spin on the tale. He spoke about how, during a lengthy career in the fire service, there are calls that will haunt us. This can be explained as a firefighter drives in the neighborhood where they work. "Over here is where we delivered that baby…On this block, we had the jumpers…Remember when we lost that homeless man to heroin over there?" The locations of these incidents will always be a snapshot in the minds of these brave men and women. I'd bet that they could walk us through every aspect of how the call unfolded, down to the very clothing the patients were wearing. These are the ghosts that are represented in this movie and in the lives of firefighters. One of the first things a firefighter will do after they have a bad call is second guess their actions. What if I sent the water quicker? What if I pushed epi sooner? What if I drove to the hospital faster? It is in our nature to challenge the facts.

My goal is to provide answers to these questions. By identifying what is amiss with someone, they can at least have some semblance of knowledge about why they feel the way they do. "Because knowing is half the battle!" (Bacal, et.al.,1983-1986). Right, *GI Joe* fans? After understanding 'why I do what it is I do,' comes the amazing part: solutions. There are vast amounts of literature on identifying mental health issues. That is all fine and dandy, but the firefighter will then ask, "What do I do about it?" This book is intended to first help identify, and then help to overcome.

Throughout this text, I have used three voices: my personal voice, my firefighter voice and my counselor voice. Each one tells a different perspective. My personal voice would be called *The Elephant*. Elephants are naturally inquisitive. They will become playful with each other, but they remain loyal to their family and friends. Elephants also endure hardships. Their tusks are widely sought after, and they must continue in life with the burden of death hanging over their heads. It is this adversity that they must conquer as they navigate their homelands. My firefighter voice would be called *The Ox*. Working hard to plow the field, oxen have no one to impress. It is due diligence and the reward of hard work that keeps them steadfast on this course. After being well fed and watered, they will work all day until sunset, with no questions asked. My counselor voice would be *The Crow*. Known to be clever, crows will fashion their own tools to accomplish a task. It is this ingenuity that allows their intelligence to shine. They are also known to recognize human faces and possess complex thoughts, like thinking about the future. The crow is pragmatic, precise, and purposeful.

It is these voices that drive this text to be woven into a tapestry of thought. Make of it what you will, but I do hope that my sincerity, my hard work, and my knowledge will be handed to you, my reader, in a way that gives credibility to the ideas I have shown. Mental health within the fire service is approaching a precipice of greatness. By instilling these values and pearls of wisdom in the next generation of firefighters, I hope to accomplish the greatest feat: making the next generation of firefighters better than that which preceded it.

WHO HELPS THE HELPERS?

"What would you do if I sang out of tune? Would you stand up and walk out on me? Lend me your ears and I'll sing you a song, and I'll try not to sing out of key. I get by with a little help from my friends."

(Lennon & McCartney, 1967)

If you ask any firefighter if they think of themselves as a hero, they will reply with an emphatic "No!" The feats these wonderful human beings perform can be over the top and often become fodder for the news media. They could rescue a child from a three-story building fire or pry a pregnant mother from a pin-in accident, but they will certainly shy away when it comes to others calling them a hero. You see, it is not the post-event response after a firefighter performs a miraculous save that becomes the impetus for their motivation. It is the act of helping others which plays a central role in their need to help others. Oftentimes, when a firefighter decides to follow the path into the fire service, it is their own prior adversity that helps them arrive at this destination. But when the cameras roll after an incident and the public or commentators tell the firefighters they are heroes, they will most certainly all reply the same way. We are not heroes. It is our training that takes over, allowing us to make the save. We are simply doing our job. This humble response, though, often directly relates to the difficulty that ensues when trying to help firefighters from a counseling perspective. When a traumatic call occurs and it affects a firefighter's mental health, they will chalk it up as just doing their job. Of course, some (unfortunately they are few and far between) go their whole careers with a stone cold constitution and never let years of service affect their mental health, but most are not able to do this. It is these individuals who can benefit most from counseling.

How can you help someone who does not want help? This is quite the conundrum for a counselor choosing to work with this population. According to the Firefighter Behavioral Health Alliance, 97 firefighters and 26 EMTs and paramedics died by suicide in 2020. This number dwarfs the amount of Line of Duty Deaths (LODD), which sits at 67 members, during the same time period (Hoban, 2021). Thus, there is definitely a need. Firefighters frequently require mental health counseling. So, how do we go about putting this pipe dream into fruition? After all, who helps the helpers when they are in need? The best way to illustrate this is to share the story of *Androcles and the Lion*.

During the times of ancient Rome, there was a slave named Androcles. He was not happy with being a slave, so he decided to run away. While he was walking through the forest, he came upon a treacherous sight. It was a *lion*! Unlike other lions, this particular one seemed quite docile and did not eat him upon greeting him. After further investigation, Androcles realized that the lion was in distress. The lion crept up to Androcles, using three of his four legs, and cowered in front of him. After further inspection, Androcles saw a thorn in the mighty animal's front paw. Carefully, so as not to scare the lion, Androcles approached him and gingerly removed the thorn from his paw. The lion was so grateful, he brought Androcles a fawn so the two of them could feast and enjoy each other's company. Shortly after this meeting, Androcles was arrested by Roman guards and was charged with running away. His punishment was to be thrown into the arena and defend himself against fantastic beasts. So, Androcles, armed with a dull spear, was positioned to fight a pack of lions. As the lions were released inside the arena, one of them cautiously approached Androcles. It was the lion that he had helped by extracting the thorn from his paw! The lion nuzzled Androcles' hand and laid at his feet. The king was in awe of this spectacle and demanded a response.

After Androcles explained the circumstances, the king set them both free. Androcles was no longer a slave, and the lion returned to the forest (Shaw, 1962).

Most firefighters will identify with Androcles. He is the underdog. He risked his life in order to help someone else, knowing that doing so would possibly put himself in danger. This is what firefighters do. They put on their uniform in the morning and expect to put their life on the line for others so that they, too, can have a second chance at life. It is a mixture of perseverance, empathy, and strength that allows them to do this, but I see it from a different perspective. I think that the firefighters are also the lion. You see, the lion is gruff, powerful and a force to be reckoned with…much like a firefighter. But, the lion did something remarkable. He sought help. He realized he could not ambulate, and this does not bode well for a lion in the forest. It was a rare and uncomfortable move, asking a human for help, but he did it. And by doing so, his problem was resolved. Firefighters, not unlike the lion, are not impervious to similar sorts of obstacles.

It is my goal as a firefighter and a counselor to reframe the generally existing view that firefighters have regarding mental health. It is okay to be Androcles and help others that are in need. But it is also okay to be the lion and accept help from others when you are no longer able to handle it by yourself. To them I say be vulnerable, be brave. Be the lion.

FROM THE BEGINNING

"Penny Lane, there is a fireman with an hourglass and in his pocket is a portrait of the Queen. He likes to keep his fire engine clean. It's a clean machine."

(Lennon & McCartney, 1967)

My department was reeling from some major issues. We had a battle with the city that positioned the department against a steadfast mayor who was deliberately avoiding the terms of our collective bargaining agreement. Our members were forced to make tough decisions, up to and including quitting the job. At the same time, we had a line of duty death (LODD) of an active member. The rank and file were reeling. In addition to this, the COVID-19 pandemic had companies working short-handed, rigs were downgraded, and mandatory overtime was rampant, keeping people away from their families. As a place to vent, people would turn to the union social media group page. In reviewing their posts, I saw my fellow co-workers in such disarray that it made me want to help. I threw my business card on the page and put a little blip about reaching out if someone is having issues. That's when the fun started.

It just so happened that a retired curmudgeon called me out on this same forum, asking such things as who I was, what my qualifications were, and even going as far as to question my intentions by calling my efforts a cash grab. Now, having more than twenty years on the job, I assumed that most members knew who I was, and because I had posted my bio prior to this, I had hoped most were in the loop. Well, I was quite wrong. However, as much as I wanted to yell from the mountaintops how I was only there to help, I realized this gentleman had something of a point. So, I penned a post, not only for him, but for all the members who might not know who I was. What I learned in this instance is, you can never assume that others know who you are or can be confident that you do not have nefarious intentions. So this is me explaining who I am to you.

Out of high school, I followed what was then the natural path of going to college and found that it was not the best fit for me. Even though I was independent and motivated, I allowed the culture of parties, dorm gatherings and newly-found freedom to get in the way of my studies. After the first year, it was quite obvious to my parents that they should not be spending one more dime on *The Adventures of Gregg: The College Years.* That summer, I begged, pleaded and even went so far as to run away from home to hammer my point forward that I wanted to stay in school. With disgust, my parents went against their better judgment and enrolled me on a probationary basis. I was sure I would not disappoint. Well, this story ends with me eating crow. I not only failed, but I had to find a way to pay my parents back for the wasted semester. I was beside myself. With no direction, no money and nothing binding me, I did what every teenage boy would do: I followed the *Grateful Dead!*

Even though the challenges of the years that followed were formidable, the time I spent reflecting on my future was wonderful. During this time, I remember hearing a friend talking about how someone she knew was a firefighter. I was dumbfounded! Someone our age was a firefighter? How can that be? I regularly asked her about his training: EMT training, the fire academy, and more. The more I consulted her about this guy, the more it resonated with me. I reflected on what it would be like if I was a firefighter helping people in their time of need. I certainly could do that. So, I mustered up every stitch of confidence I had and marched into my hometown municipal firehouse and squeaked, "Hello Sir, I wanna be a firefighter." Looking back now, I would love to speak with the chap that handled this exchange. It would be priceless! This man endearingly told me that they were not hiring right now, and he suggested that I go to the next town over, since they were a volunteer fire department. After going to this second place, I began the process: applications, interviews, and more applications followed by more interviews. Ultimately, I got a phone call late one night. They told me I was hired, with the stipulation that I would cut my hair, shave my beard and go into the fire academy. I was going to be a firefighter!

The schooling was swift. I would be hired full-time; however, I had set my sights higher. I wanted to be a Chicago firefighter! The CFD had opened the list for paramedics in 1998, and I got called to report to the Quinn Fire Academy on August 1, 2001. I ended up on an ambulance in the Austin neighborhood of Chicago where we did, on average, 18 to 22 calls in a 24-hour period. It was vastly different from the two to three calls we were doing in my sleepy suburban job previously. And, boy, did I cut my teeth. I covered every trauma and medical patient that my standing medical orders allowed me to do. After eight years of service as a paramedic, I finally got the call to process and become a firefighter. I would go back to the academy, this time to learn about such things as building construction, forcing a door, and leading out a fire hose. I was green, but I was motivated and humble. As time went on, my seniority built and I was able to go back to the same firehouse at which I had been a paramedic. Only this time, I was on the engine. And then it happened…

There was definitely a cohort of us. We all joined at about the same time. We all went on dates together. Eventually, some of us got married around the same time, and then the children followed. All of life's benchmarks were happening before our very eyes. I remember waking up one particular morning, though, and receiving a phone call that our friend Chris was dead. He had died the night before at a restaurant fire. My wife, being an emergency room nurse at the time, had known Chris even before I did when they both worked in the suburbs. We were beside ourselves. To this day, one of the hardest things I have had to do was to let Chris' friend, who was now a firefighter in Texas, know of Chris' passing. My wife insisted I do it personally, and it was the right thing to do. We didn't know what to do, so we got dressed and went to Chris' firehouse. There was a large gathering there of family, friends and co-workers trickling in after hearing of his passing. Chris was gone, and there was nothing that we could do to change that.

A couple days later, I received a call from a friend's wife. She made me aware that her husband was having a real hard time dealing with the loss of our friend. My wife and I invited the two of them over to process the grief. We laughed, we cried, we got mad, and we hugged. It was cathartic for all of us. As the days unfolded, there were more and more people that wanted to talk. People needed an outlet and didn't know where to turn. This would become a turning point for me in determining what I would do next. It would, in fact, forever change the trajectory of my life.

It just so happened that the CFD, the third largest fire department (behind only New York and LA County), had a minimalistic view of mental health issues and their rank-and-file. There were a total of two clinicians to serve approximately 5,000 members. *Two!* On the other hand, the union did have a grass-roots program that aimed to help those in need; however, no one involved in the program had any formal education in how to deal with the intricacies of first responders and their mental health issues. I spoke with my wife and told her I wanted to go back to school and become a counselor. I saw the writing on the wall. In the immortal words of Mahatma Gandhi, "If we could change ourselves, the tendencies in the world would also change. As a man changes his own nature, so does the attitude of the world change towards him...We need not wait to see what others do" (Gandhi, 1999, p. 241). After all, I was a firefighter and a paramedic. Who would better understand what my peers were going through than a counselor with those similar credentials? I had been in the trenches. I understood the schedule, the lack of sleep, the danger, and the hundreds of other challenges. I recall multiple times where I held a fatally wounded child in my hands. I knew what it was like to not know how I got home in the morning due to being so extremely tired from being up all night running calls. But where would I begin?

Since I had virtually no usable undergraduate credits to my name (I don't think badminton and underwater basket weaving counted towards a degree), I enrolled at Penn State University in a program called World Campus. Being a virtual program, it would allow me to continue to work at the fire department as well as attend two to three classes a semester. The irony was that the only time I saw the campus was when I graduated, with my wife and parents watching from the stands and beaming as I walked across the stage. (Thanks be to God, no one else knew that I almost tripped on the last step of the riser after I received my diploma!) I took the summer off of work that year and began my graduate training at Concordia University in clinical mental health counseling. Would you know it? I graduated top of my class with a 4.0! Things were certainly looking up for me.

I was blessed to then have an internship at a group practice where I would be able to hone my craft of treating first responders in both an individual and couples capacity. After my internship was up, I spoke with my director and she said a job was mine if I wanted it. Oh, I wanted it! My director and I devised a strategy to get people in for therapy. She asked me if I remembered the TV show *M*A*S*H**. I responded with a resounding, "Duh! It was one of my favorites!" She asked if I remembered the psychologist on the show that was just out of view and happened to be at the right place at the right time when the soldiers needed assistance with their mental health. "Major Sidney Freedman!," I promptly responded. Since I was immersed in the firehouse already, I could act as a guide to steer those that were in need. It was a brilliant plan! (Gelbart, 1972-1983).

However, I soon found out how messed up our rank-and-file really was. Alcoholism, drug abuse, sex addiction and rampant gambling were just a few of the issues that were prevalent among my colleagues. I would float around the city and, after dinner, I would grab a cup of coffee. Many of us would sit around the rigs, campfire style, and talk about how to solve the world's problems. I would use this as my opportunity to get a pulse on how everyone was doing mentally. More often than not, people would spill: about a bad call, about their family life, about their emotions, about what they might do to combat all of these issues and many others. I would try to offer a bit of knowledge about anger management and self-care, whatever I could offer, and after explaining my role as a therapist, I would hand them my card.

Once the ball began to roll, my work became busier, and I realized how badly what I had to offer was needed. After all, these individuals are immersed in an occupation that absolutely requires being a part of some very bad situations. For example, if two cars crash into each other and there are at least five patients, we call this a *Plan 1*. To the general public, it would be a flurry of carnage and chaos. To first responders, this is where we are in our happy place. Picture the movie *The Matrix* with Keanu Reeves. When he jumps up in a graceful, calculated way to karate kick his opponent, the world seems to freeze. All sides are now visible to him and he becomes one with the moment (Wachowski & Wachowski,1999). It is a very Zen-like response to an extremely stressful situation. That is how we, as first responders, respond. We are better, sometimes, at controlling chaos. We then bring the stories of these calls back to the firehouse and they are repeated to the next shift, through the battalion, and so on. When I first got on the department, I quickly learned that lay people did not really want to hear about the calls we went on, even though they often asked what the worst call I have been on was. I remember telling them about the four-year-old that fell out of a second story window, or the lady that was pinned against a store by a car and when we got to her, there wasn't much left of her legs. The reactions I would get to these stories made it clear to me that people don't really want to hear about what we see. They feign interest, but they sincerely do not want to know. So, that leaves us to carry the burden.

Ultimately, the onus falls on us to make changes in our lives. It is easier to bitch and complain about *not* having services for our members. It just so happens that helping others is in my wheelhouse. Being a certified, card-carrying member of the empath club, I find it fulfilling and natural to talk to people about what works and what doesn't. Whether it's finding ways to elevate one's coping skills or getting to the root of why someone is angry with every fiber in their body, it is my goal to try and tackle mental health in a positive, non-judgmental, and confidential manner. My situation is unique. Being entrenched in the mix, meaning that I work at the fire department one day and I see the same people in my office a day later in a therapeutic manner, I must hold confidentiality to a premium. I tell my clients that if someone finds out about them going to counseling, it was not from me. If I did not strenuously maintain confidentiality, I would not have a practice. But eventually something magical started to happen. The people I saw in therapy who pleaded that no one find out about them seeing me, became the same people that are now normalizing therapy to their family and friends. Regularly, I hear them going out into the community and telling people that they are seeing their therapist – of their own accord! These clients are my biggest advocates, and they are the reason I have a constant flow of referrals.

Looking back at this journey, I feel like I am blessed. I get to do a job that people write into movies. Meanwhile, I also have the opportunity to help important and at-risk people with their mental health issues. It truly is a dual role. Firefighter/Paramedic Gregg Bagdade, Licensed Professional Counselor. It has a nice ring to it. So, to that retired curmudgeon, I thank you, for you taught me that we must always start off from the beginning.

NO, REALLY, I'M FINE

"Everywhere people stare each and every day. I can see them laugh at me, and I hear them say. 'Hey! You've got to hide your love away.'"

(Lennon & McCartney, 1965)

I have a simple, go-to tactic I use when encouraging people to take care of their mental health. I'll ask, "If you were on a call and you lacerated your hand, what would you do?" The respondent would probably answer nervously with something like, "I would ask the medic to butterfly it because I don't want to go on medical roll." After the two of us share a chuckle, I then dig deeper. I would introduce a more dastardly injury, such as a degloved finger or an open ankle fracture. More often than not, their demeanor changes and the retort is less dismissively humorous; they'll say, "I would go to the emergency room." Once this recognition of relative severity is established, albeit in a roundabout way, I try to explain that experiencing a traumatic event will have a detrimental, and potentially lasting effect on a person's life. The brain's chemistry adjusts accordingly, and the physiological effects can disrupt someone's life, making work, social, and family relationships difficult to navigate. Trauma is trauma. Whether it is a soft tissue/skeletal injury or an injury to someone's mental health, it needs to be addressed by a professional. Period.

13

So, why is it that the laceration will be taken care of professionally, but having insomnia and constantly replaying thoughts about a call where a child was in a bad car accident will be thrown by the wayside? If you ask a hundred firefighters why this is so, most of them will brush it off for one main reason: they do not want to be looked at any differently by their peers. This negative stigma enveloping issues with mental health runs deep within the fire service.

In fact, this stigma really begins during the hiring process. In order to become a firefighter, there are a battery of tests the applicant must take, both written and physical. There are some places that require oral interviews as well as psychological exams (which, for the most part, are limited to personality assessments). The hiring fire department will make a list of the candidates and rank them utilizing criteria that ensures those with the highest scores are hired first. After they are hired, these new candidates will enter a fire academy. Again, their success and forward progression will depend on didactic and physical scores. This conundrum continues throughout the candidate's career, as they must take promotional exams to elevate their pay as well as their position within the fire department.

The problem with this promotion culture is that it discourages anyone from being or even appearing less than perfect. Throughout a typical candidate's career, they are *literally* told that they have to be the best or they will not succeed. During a recent visit to a firehouse, I watched as a seasoned Captain, with more fire experience than most will ever see in their career, took our candidate aside to give him some pearls of wisdom. I hung around to listen. Within an hour and a half of listening to the Captain bestow his information on us, we were beaming with knowledge. At this time, I had more than 20 years of experience, many of these in low socioeconomic status (SES) neighborhoods, giving me an education within the school of hard knocks. But, as an old timer once told me early in my career, the moment you know it all is the moment you must retire. This is because you become a liability to yourself and others, since nobody will ever truly be able to know everything there is to know about a topic. Someone will surely get hurt as a result. Later in the day, my candidate and I were talking about the process of learning throughout one's career. I said that a person with five or six years on the job would not ask for help on a subject since it would, in his view, show weakness. People would rather not know how to do something than admit that they cannot do it. This was reflected by the fact that, in a house of twelve firefighters, we were the only ones attending this impromptu training session. It was kind of sad.

This translates directly within the realm of mental health. I would like to imagine a world where, after a high acuity call, the members were debriefed and, if necessary, encouraged to seek individual counseling. But this is only a dream! The reality of the situation is that members would much more likely go back to the firehouse after putting themselves back in service, eat their meal that's now cold, and continue to go on more calls as required by our job description until the end of their tour of duty. I once asked a chief what he does to check on his members' mental health after a call. His response was primitive. He would ask his crew if they were all good. Something is better than nothing, I suppose, but let's dissect this.

Let's say John and Mary went on a call where an older gentleman was living in utter squalor. There were rats, cockroaches and maggots galore. Living as he did among the veritable zoo of vermin and insects, this man was severely malnourished and unkempt. After the crew prepared him for transport, he went into full arrest and his heart stopped. Even though the crew tried valiantly to resuscitate this man to the best of their ability, he did not make it. Afterward, John continued to think about the call as he climbed into his bunk. It so happened that he had a father that was in a similar situation. Although his father was not in squalor, he was suffering from cancer and was extremely frail, requiring much medical attention. Days after this call, John continued to obsessively think about this man and relate it to his father's situation.

John is most likely going to suppress his difficulty digesting this. Why? Because of stigma. He does not want to be considered weak or a liability by his peers or superiors. John has worked very hard to get to the point where he is today. He got hired, went through the academy (top of his class), and now he is an officer. What would the others think of him if he, an award- winning veteran of the fire service, had issues dealing with a call? After getting back to the firehouse, the chief stops by quarters and the three of them talk about this call in a very benign and sterile way. "You all good?" the chief asks, knowing that John had an ill father. John responds, "Yeah, I'm good, Chief." He feels this is the only response he could give. If only he had twisted his ankle on the run, then perhaps he would have gotten the help he needed.

On the other hand, if John chose instead to receive counseling, he would be better able to process why he is bothered by this call and to connect the dots with the dim situation his father is in. But he won't. He won't because he feels that, by having an issue, he becomes a liability to his fellow members. He feels that the other people in his firehouse will judge him. He feels that he is weak for having these issues. He feels others will think he is not able to do the job to his best ability and that they will not be able to depend on him in a difficult situation. In a career where competition is at a premium, it is unacceptable to have a chink in one's armor. But why is this situation not held to the same standard as the twisted ankle? Is it because we can see the ankle and thus know that the person actually has a physical deficit that affects his ability to work? Instead, John will continue to suffer emotionally, push it down and go on to the next call, and the next, and the next.

I've been asked how we can improve mental health awareness within the fire service, and my answer is always the same: Attrition. The old timers who seek counseling, if they even do, will do it under duress. They have been served divorce papers, they get a DWI, they commit battery, or they have lost a large amount of money due to high-risk gambling. It is then that they become *re*active and try to get help. More often than not, these individuals will want a "quick fix" which will, in their minds, equate to only a couple sessions. This simply isn't practical. Those that go to counseling know quite well that it may take months, if not years, to do the work and get resolve from the adversity that one may endure.

It is the younger generation of firefighters that carry the torch, putting mental health awareness in a positive light. They are much more in tune with introspection, processing emotional fortitude, and being able to put in the work weekly to get their ills from their head space to their mouth space. I often use this vernacular to describe what it means to get the thought, emotion, or event out of their mind and expel it by speaking about it. The aftermath of a traumatic event can be extremely taxing on a firefighter or paramedic. The days that follow the event are troublesome because these individuals will try to navigate their days as if nothing remarkable has happened. But, consequently, the more they try to compartmentalize, the more they will have issues. They may chew on the incident, reliving it over and over. Talking about the incident with a trained professional would be ideal, but simply expelling the baggage to a safe confidant can be just as therapeutic. Dr. Gabor Maté, one of the premier psychologists on trauma and addiction says it like this, "No society can understand itself without looking at its shadow side" (Maté, 2018, p.2). It is these younger members who will normalize going to a counselor, setting the table for others to get the help they so desperately need.

When the general public envisions what a firefighter looks like, they are immediately drawn to the chisel jawed, stubble faced men, or the make-up faced, perfectly coiffed women that they see on television or in the movies. It is these types that will arrive when I have my emergency and call 9-1-1 to help me through the worst day of my life. But, along with the image that people have of these first responders, comes the idea that they can handle any situation mentally, regardless of the magnitude. Because, why not? They chose this profession. They should be able to deal with anything, right? What is missing from the public's assessment can be spoken in three words...*they are human*. The people that come to your house live in a community not unlike yours. They are mothers and sons. Little league coaches and PTO representatives. When you need a ladder to clean your gutters, they are next door to supply one and be the first to ask if you need help. But, most importantly, firefighters are *human*! People forget that. When I began in the fire service, I remember trying to avoid looking at the family photos on the wall when I had to tell them their loved one was deceased and we did all we could do. We are taught in paramedic school to look at a patient as if they are a vehicle engine and assess the situation in a logical, yet expeditious manner. By doing this, it takes away a small part of empathy that we might have for them – a sort of disconnect. But, when my eyes would go adrift from the patient, I'd often scan the room; sometimes I would see the family photos, and there was the patient, all smiles, surrounded by their loved ones. I'd be lying if I told you I didn't get a little misty eyed. Why would that happen? Because I am human. Because I have a heart. We all share that same empathy or else we would not have gone into this field. What would happen if I did show emotion to this particular family? To most, it is not welcome. First responders are there to help the public when they are in a dire situation. Save lives and property, right?

I remember seeing the movie *Patton* with George C. Scott playing the namesake. The movie took place during World War II and portrayed the life of George S. Patton, a United States General who was stern, strict, and no nonsense. During one scene, General Patton visited a military hospital that was caring for wounded men from the battlefield. He knelt down next to one soldier in particular and inquired about his situation. The soldier replied that he was tired of the shelling and he could no longer take it. General Patton's response was overly aggressive. He began yelling at the soldier and hitting him in the helmet with his gloves. He ordered the soldier to be returned to the front lines immediately and called him a coward (Schaffner, F.J., 1970). I am not a veteran. I was always envious of those that served. To this day, I make sure myself and my family thank the brave veterans that served our country to maintain our freedom. I am not saying that the atrocities of war don't far outweigh those seen within the fire service. I am simply trying to draw a parallel to what they both see. A traumatic event is a traumatic event. It is okay to have it affect you.

There are plenty of people within the ranks of the fire service that would, to this very day, respond in a very similar fashion to a member that was overcome with emotion after a traumatic call. I doubt there would be physical violence and name calling, but the sentiment would surely be there. In their eyes, it is simply not okay to be not okay. So, how do we change this? What is the best way to allow our members to be not okay?

WE ARE NOT MEANT TO SEE THIS...

"He blew his mind out in a car. He didn't notice that the lights had changed. A crowd of people stood and stared."

(Lennon & McCartney, 1967)

Prior to getting on the city, I worked in a sleepy suburb of Chicago that was known for its downtown area. It looked like a veritable Christmas village, and last I heard they filmed a Hallmark Channel Christmas Special there. I guess if the shoe fits, right? What a great start I got from this volunteer fire department, though. I was coming off of an adventure that Jack Kerouac would have been proud of, but now it was time to get down to brass tacks. I was such a mess. I didn't know about such basics as hygiene, making a bed, and coming to work in a punctual manner. The firefighters that I worked with made me their pet project and decided to work with me. Their diligence created the man I am today. The paramilitary structure that the fire service provided was the impetus I needed to get the ball rolling for my career and my life. I am forever thankful to the members of the Long Grove Fire Protection District for giving a scrub like myself a chance at a wonderful career.

But, the leap I made from this suburban oasis to the mean streets of Chicago catapulted me more than I could ever have imagined. I entered the academy for the Chicago Fire Department on day one at 0700 hours – squared away as best as I could be. I got my city address (the Chicago Fire Department has a residency requirement) and my proper documentation showing that I was a paramedic in good standing with the State of Illinois. I had a thirst for knowledge to learn things The Chicago Way.

"Candidate Paramedic Bagdade! Please stand up!" shouted the commander of the academy.

"Candidate Paramedic Bagdade is present and accounted for!" I retorted, standing at attention.

The commander briefly stated, "You are dismissed. Medical will contact you."

I was dumbfounded – at an absolute loss. Not knowing what was going on, I reported to the medical division. After speaking with them, it was clear they had very little to say. Was I dying? Was I okay? Was someone in my family dying? What was the reason for my dismissal? The drive home involved a lot of anger, swearing, hitting the steering wheel, and ugly crying. I soon received a letter from the medical division stating that they wanted paperwork from my doctor that said I would not swear at the people I was taking care of since I had Tourette's Syndrome. Tourette's Syndrome is a central nervous system disorder that involves nervous tics and involuntary movements, including something called coprolalia, which is uncontrolled swearing or cursing. I began to laugh! My Tourette's had been quite under control ever since my doctors found the correct dose of medication for me. This occurred when I was seven years old. No one really knows that I have Tourette's unless I disclose it to them. After I secured the appropriate paperwork, I was good to go. I was thrust into the academy.

A month in, we were learning about High Rise Incident Command when our instructor brought a large television on a cart with wheels into the classroom. He turned on the news. It was the World Trade Center in New York City. One of the buildings had thick black smoke pouring out of a floor very high up. And then it happened…BAM! The second plane hit the other tower. Up to this point, we thought we were watching a high rise fire and expected the boys and girls of the FDNY to make a quick stop, but this was entirely different. We sat watching the whole thing unfold with feelings of helplessness. When the first tower fell, the pit in my stomach became a nauseating manifestation of the grief I felt for those poor souls in that building. Then the instructor spoke chilling words...

"I'd like to turn off the television right now, if that's okay. To think that in a matter of minutes, I just lost a hundred friends."

Friends...he was talking about firefighters! Before we knew it, we were marching to the drill yard. Chief Chikerotis, a legend on CFD and now a consultant for the TV show *Chicago Fire*, approached us. "Everyone, take a knee." We were told that America was under attack and we could be next. He then asked if any of us were firefighters in the suburbs before we got on. Myself and about five other people raised their hands. "Good!" He was enthused, "You all go load hose into the spare engines while the rest of the medics bring supplies into the spare ambulances." For those that remember, all American aircrafts were grounded until further notice. So, there we were, a minute on the job, loading hose on *real* CFD engines in full view of the Sears Tower. Occasionally, a plane would fly overhead and it would end up being a military plane doing their rounds, but the silence was deafening (minus the afterburners helping them tear through the sky like warrior birds). When all was said and done, Chicago did not get attacked, and I returned to my studio apartment unscathed but thinking, *What in the world did I get myself into?*

After my momentous start, I turned toward being the best paramedic I could be. I would say that I definitely cut my teeth on the west side of Chicago. I was stationed at Ambulance 23 out of Engine 113's house in the South Austin neighborhood. When the general public thinks of violent crime in Chicago, they think of two neighborhoods: Englewood (on the south side) and Austin (on the west side). Austin was unique in that it was right near the Eisenhower Expressway (affectionately dubbed The Heroin Highway because of its convenience for people from all over the Chicago metropolitan area to come in, get their heroin, and bolt back to the suburbs). Due to this open market drug trading, there were constant turf wars fought on the city streets between gangs trying to establish dominance. This was often done through gun violence.

To put it bluntly, I do not remember a shift where we didn't have at least one gunshot victim. Sometimes it was one. Sometimes it was eight. We got really good at caring for these victims and keeping them stable until we could bring them to a Level I Trauma Center. During the Gulf War, we had Army medics ride with us so they could get trauma experience before going into battle. During this time, I saw our patients, grown men, pleading for their lives. Regularly, they would ask for their mommas. Who wouldn't in their ultimate time of need? You see, we were not there to judge, and we certainly were not the jury. We were there to help these people in their most desperate time of need. It was *literally* a matter of life and death! When we pulled up to the scene, there was nothing that my suburban job could have prepared me for. Among the screaming and crying, there were police telling us who was shot. There were family members and friends yelling at me to treat their loved ones, not understanding that the gray matter coming out of their half-blown head was incident enough for us to not work them. But we did. We saved a lot. We also lost a lot. Sometimes, we would get patients that were so badly shot, they were brain dead. This meant that they no longer had any brain activity, but their heart was still beating. "Why are we treating these patients? There's no hope for them," the medics would ask. I would tell them, "We may not be able to save them, but their beating heart, as well as their other organs, will let someone else live another day." If anything, our efforts would not go to waste.

About seven years later, I crossed the floor to become a cross-trained firefighter paramedic. This involved going back to the academy to learn how to be a firefighter. After some time on the street after the academy, I transferred to the same house where I had been a medic. Only this time, I was on the engine. The way CFD structures their calls is that my engine was an Advanced Life Support (ALS) engine staffed by me (a medic) and an EMT, at minimum. We would respond to EMS calls as either a support to the ambulance, or when there was not an ambulance close by. My engine would arrive first to render care until the next closest ambulance could arrive. Because I was a medic, I had a full complement of ALS supplies at my disposal: a drug box full of medications, IV fluids, intubation supplies, and a cardiac monitor, with a defibrillator, to analyze their heart rhythm. I also had access to many basic life-saving supplies such as tourniquets, splints, gauze bandages, obstetrical kits, and more. Of course, we would also respond to any fire related incident as well.

At times when someone in our still district (our area that we covered) got shot and the ambulance transported the patient to the hospital, my engine would then respond back to the incident to do what is called a washdown. A washdown consists of taking a firehose and a scrub brush and simply washing the blood and guts off the concrete, making sure it goes down the sewer drain. I assure you, if this was not done, the streets of Austin would surely be running red with the blood of its residents. One time, my crew was dispatched to a call exactly like this. We were just finishing up our housework prior to this and everyone was feeling jovial. We got out of the rig, grabbed our necessary tools, and began deluging the human matter down the drain. Some of the guys were laughing and busting each other's stones as they completed the task. I looked around and saw all sorts of people from the neighborhood gathering. There were neighbors, family members, and some of them were children. This was not the spectacle I wanted to be a part of. I told the guys curtly to, "Cut it out!" and gestured to them that we were being inappropriate. After looking at the neighborhood folk, I soon realized that what we were doing had a *large* impact on this dilapidated area.

But, you see? That's just it. For firefighters, it simply becomes routine to be present for the macabre. It is no secret that people in the fire service have a dark sense of humor. After all, it is the defense mechanism of choice that allows us to be present for such disturbing incidents. Can you even imagine John Q Public handling the resuscitation of a child that just recently choked on a hotdog and is now breathing? Can you now imagine the situation if the child, even after all of your life saving maneuvers, did not survive? How does one deal with that? Most first responders, both urban and rural, have experienced these horrors, among many others, and returned to work as if nothing had happened.

At the time of this writing, I am stationed at Engine 26/Truck 7/ Ambo 45. Our firehouse is closest to the Cook County Morgue. When auto accidents happen on one of the expressways and someone involved in the accident dies in the car but are unretrievable, the tow truck brings the car and the entrapped person to the morgue for further investigation. They routinely then call Truck 7 to cut this person out. The guys come back and talk about how gross the patients were...eyeballs bulging out, intestines exposed. On one such occasion, a firefighter told me that a younger girl was burned beyond recognition, and both her legs were fractured when the dashboard hit her. He recalled the smell of her burning flesh, as well as the torment she must have gone through while being entrapped in this fiery tomb.

These are the real horrors brought on by the trade that so many of us revere. It is these scenes and the experiences that go with them that shape how we continue on with life. Some firefighters will not be fazed by these atrocities. They will simply go on with life and continue to be quite well adjusted. Others will act out in various ways...through drinking, gambling, anger, high risk sexual activity, the list of maladaptive coping mechanisms is unlimited. Our goal as counselors is to rest assured that all members go home to their families and have a happy, healthy, well-adjusted life. But, it needs to be recognized that the amount of horrors that firefighters see every day is astronomical. It is they that must harbor these scenes and simply move on to the next call. Most refuse to believe this, but they must carry this cross throughout their whole career.

MORE TRAUMA THAN DRAMA

"Boy, you're gonna carry that weight, carry that weight for a long time."

(Lennon & McCartney, 1968)

Since I began my counseling practice with the intent of having first responders as my population of choice, I needed to get buy-in from the very people that I would be treating. I began by going to suburban fire departments and presenting to them. The presentations were designed for me to talk about my career and have them understand that I was not unlike them at all. After 20 years of service with the Chicago Fire Department, I had seen some very horrific calls. It was my aim to gain favor by placing myself in their shoes. *Empathy.* Empathy is such a powerful tool that counselors can use to show a client that we not only hurt for the victim, but we understand what they are going through. It doesn't take a numbskull to understand that a counselor saying, "I'm sorry you went through that," is not as valid as them saying, "I'm sorry you went through that. I get it. I've been there."

Another key point that I try to make is that counselors are not superior to the client. Just because the client is seeking professional help from the counselor, it does not mean that they are any better than them. As students, we are taught to develop rapport with the client. This may be done immediately, or it may take some time, depending on the individual. The important thing is to make the client feel comfortable enough to want to share their innermost secrets with you. They are vulnerable, a raw nerve. Yet, there is no ranking structure here. Within the fire service, there is a paramilitary organization that must be followed. The subordinates report to their Lieutenant, the Lieutenant reports to a Battalion Chief, and so on through the chain. When someone is suffering from mental health issues, it is important that we break this chain of command. Positive mental health is superior to any ranking structure available to us. I cannot begin to say how many times I have learned about myself from one of my clients. I have found several times that I took the advice of a client because it appeared to be a prudent suggestion. We are equal. The same playing field.

One of the first stories I tell is of a fiery car crash my company responded to. We were dispatched to an auto fire. When we arrived, we found a sedan that had run into a light pole. There were several people that had gotten ejected from the vehicle strewn about. Some had lost limbs or parts of appendages. But one woman was still in the vehicle. I led out the firehose and waited for the water. As I waited, I saw this woman struggling to get out of the vehicle, but because of the extensive damage to the automobile, it was futile for her to get out. The flames grew and grew. My waiting for the water to fill my hose seemed like an eternity, even though it was merely minutes in real time. The woman was engulfed in the flames as she banged on the window to get out. My Lieutenant took his Halligan bar, shattered the window and reached in to pull her out, but the flames were too much for him. When I eventually got water to my hose, I attacked the fire with all the gusto I could muster. We were going to save this woman just in time! When the dust settled, and the fire was put out, the ambulance pulled the woman out of the car. She looked like one of those CPR mannequins, with no distinguishing features. The burns were so extensive, she was unrecognizable, but she was breathing! Being a paramedic, I hopped into the ambulance and we treated her the best we could, taking her to Stroger Hospital (formerly Cook County Hospital) and released her to the ED staff.

When I met with my crew at the hospital, they were all beside themselves. The engineer said, "I should have sent the water quicker." The hydrant guy said, "I should have tried to force the door." The officer, now applying Silvadene ointment to his burned hands said, "I should have pulled her out...but the flames..." I went home after shift and, since it was a weekend, my wife was in bed. I woke her up. Now, my wife is a nurse. It has been very helpful having her in my life, especially when situations like this rear their ugly heads. I told her about the call. I was worried about my crew. I would have to call them to make sure they were alright. I had plans. I was in full counselor mode. My wife wasn't hearing any of it. "Gregg!" she spoke loudly. The next words out of her mouth were more pragmatic than I had expected, and it was exactly what I needed. "How can you care for others if you cannot care for yourself?" I paused in disbelief. After all, she was correct. That night, I did something that I am not particularly proud of. I met up with some old high school friends and drank a fifth of whiskey. After all, this trauma thing was relatively new to me.

Back to my presentation. I explain to my audience that the days that followed were quite riveting. I remember, particularly, going to a cosmetic shop with my wife and feeling numb. The normalcy of the shopping experience was what tipped the scales toward the abnormal. I remember thinking that this is what members of the military must go through after they come back from combat. As I write this, I feel a bit queasy because I dislike comparing wartime trauma with civilian trauma. But, even though I place our military on a pedestal, I know deep down that trauma is trauma. From the overseas battles in Kirkuk, to the mean streets of Chicago, to a spouse getting beaten regularly by their significant other. Trauma is trauma.

Soon, I found that unusual things began happening to me. First and foremost, the woman's face that we took care of, all burned and featureless, began to creep into my head. I would see her when I woke up. I would see her when I went to sleep. I would see her in my bowl of cheerios as I sat quietly at my dining room table eating breakfast. The next thing I noticed was I was having horrible nightmares. I would wake up suddenly from a quiet slumber and envision the worst things imaginable. I then noticed that I was easily startled. My daughter got me good many times when I was walking down the hallway of our home. "What, Dad? I didn't mean it!" my daughter said sheepishly as she was met with a disgruntled scowl from yours truly. Something was happening to me. My mind was stuck and I did not know how to combat this.

It doesn't take a rocket scientist to know that something was going on in my head. If you consult the DSM-5, a diagnostic manual used by mental health professionals, it seems that my symptoms were not uncommon for people who experienced a traumatic event. Intrusive thoughts? *Check.* Recurring dreams? *Check.* Flashbacks? *Check.* Irritable behavior, problems concentrating, and hypervigilance? Man! They had me pegged! These are the hallmark signs of Posttraumatic Stress Disorder (PTSD) (American Psychiatric Association, 2020). I now knew that there was a reason why I was experiencing these things. I then read the book, *The Body Keeps the Score*, by Dr. Bessel van der Kolk. He is the premier expert on anything trauma related, and I strongly urge you to read his book. As I read it, I did a lot of head nodding. He explains the brain chemistry of why this happens. In a nutshell, when someone experiences a traumatic event, their brain gets stuck in the fight/flight/freeze response. This is what happened when our ancestors would stumble upon a bear while casually picking berries. They would go into this response and do one of three things: Attempt to kill the bear, run away from the bear, or stand perfectly still so as not to seem like a threat. The problem for people who experience trauma is that their brains, particularly in the amygdala where this occurs, cannot turn off this response. Their mind continually feels that they are in danger, even when they are not. The prefrontal cortex, the front portion of the brain, is known as the gatekeeper of information. Its job, among other things, is to filter information and deem it either necessary or frivolous and act accordingly. In people who have PTSD there is a disconnect between the amygdala and the prefrontal cortex. They simply aren't communicating appropriately. So, they are stuck in this state of readiness even when the threat is averted. The results are a bevy of symptoms that are the hallmarks of PTSD (van der Kolk, 2014).

An interesting notion is that within the DSM-5, PTSD is diagnosed if certain criteria are met and the symptoms last longer than 30 days. So what happens if someone has these symptoms and it lasts less than 30 days? This is referred to as Acute Stress Disorder (ASD). The *same* criteria that is used to diagnose PTSD is also transposed to the ASD diagnosis minus the simple fact that ASD occurs up to 30 days and then resolves. I firmly believe that within the vast amount of first responders across this nation, there are far more members that have experienced ASD without fully having PTSD. Make no mistake, ASD is just as real as PTSD and the people that suffer from it need guidance in a very bad way; however, the window of opportunity to help these individuals diminishes as time goes on (2020).

A counselor's goal is to provide intervention, ideally after the traumatic event happens but before the 30 days of ASD is up. There are a multitude of ways that this can happen. In my situation, I consulted the CFD Chaplain. I chose to speak with Rabbi Moishe Wolf, the Jewish chaplain for both the Chicago Police and Fire Departments. He is a man revered in many circles. Known for telling stories to attain a life lesson or simply to explain the unexplainable, he was certainly someone that could help me in my time of need. I must specify that I did not choose him for his religious congruence, I chose him because I felt the biggest connection with him over our Protestant and Catholic affiliates. The lesson here is simply to find the help you need that fits you best. The key is to *do it*. Rabbi Wolf was not only approachable, but he was humble. I came to him to rationalize the *why* of this call. Why did she have to die? Why weren't we able to open that door? Why couldn't we extinguish the flames in time? The Rabbi set out to explain the unexplainable. He sincerely shocked me when he told me, "Gregg, death did her a favor," for the suffering she would have had to endure would not only have been excruciating, but might not have end well anyway. I know he illustrated this idea with a colorful allegory, but at the time, I was grieving. He finished the conversation by making a point to check in with me a month or two later. This is important: the follow-up. He knew that the road ahead of me would be rocky. By ensuring that I would speak with him again, he could assess and see if I would need any additional help.

Counselors know that a client must be treated at the appropriate level of care. It's kind of like taking a trauma patient to an Acute Care Center. That person would not get the optimum care due to them. This is because an Acute Care Center is not equipped with the staff, tools, and credentials to take care of said trauma patient. In the mental health world, the lowest level of care would be *individual counseling*. This is usually a weekly (sometimes bi-weekly) occurrence where the client will go to the counselor's office and the practitioner will use talk therapy to get to the bottom of what ails their client. This could last from 8-10 sessions to years, depending on what needs to be worked on. The highest level of care is *residential*. This is where the clients stay at a facility for an agreed upon time. Individual and Group therapy are used in conjunction with medications. There is much more structure and the client is overseen by professionals of multiple disciplines.

Within the fire service, these same levels of care can be applied in much the same way. A well-trained Peer Support Group can act as the initial buffer for someone that has experienced a traumatic event. I look at this as the tourniquet on the arterial bleed. By dispatching the Peer Support team, the individual(s) can decompress and talk to someone who *gets it*. The Peer Supporter is not there to *fix* the issue; they are simply there to listen. I remember seeing TV shows such as *CHiPS* (Rosner, 1977-1983) and *Emergency!* (Webb, et.al., 1972-1977) when I was young, and after a house fire or some other horrible event, the victims were given a blanket to cover themselves up with. The blanket does many things: It provides security, warmth, and protection. The Peer Support Team is there to provide these exact things. They are the initial comfort so the individual does not feel like they have to weather the storm on their own.

If the issues continue to manifest in someone's life, usually presenting as irritability, anger, or frustration, a more aggressive treatment should be considered. Oftentimes, their life becomes disrupted. They become withdrawn at work, or they lash out very easily at their family. This is where counseling should be considered, because the clinician will be able to find the reason why the individual has a disruption in their life and will know what to work on with them. A good clinician will assess the client, provide a treatment plan, and have the ability to do such things as develop a support system, teach proper coping mechanisms, encourage self-care and, among other things, find ways to deal with symptoms of the trauma such as mindfulness meditation and grounding techniques.

One particular method in the fight against ASD and PTSD is a widely researched therapy called Eye Movement Desensitization Reprocessing (EMDR). This was primarily developed by Dr. Francine Shapiro in the mid-1980s to combat the response people have when they experience trauma. Her findings teach that when we experience trauma, the incident is placed in a corrupt file within our brains. It is the goal to access this file through bilateral stimulation (BLS) and bring the distress level of this incident down to a minimum, virtually erasing it from our cognitive selves. BLS is a process in which a person will track the clinician's fingers with their eyes in a back and forth motion, left to right, over and over again. There are other techniques that are used to accomplish this, including tapping one's feet, using devices that buzz alternately in someone's hands, and more, but the goal is always the same. The goal is for the stimuli to cross from one side of the brain to the other. This is the same technique that our own body uses to process information while we sleep, commonly known as Rapid Eye Movement (REM). After the corrupt file is diminished or eliminated, the clinician will then put a positive adaptive belief (or something the client finds productive and emotionally healthy) into the file and return it to the brain. My personal experience with EMDR is not only extraordinary, but it is amazingly useful in my toolbox as I treat first responders and the trauma that they experience regularly. There are times when a couple sessions of EMDR will do the trick, and there are others that require much more comprehensive treatment in order to tackle all that is encompassing the client's issues. The analogy I use with them is that EMDR is like a sponge. If I were to take a dropper and put one drop of water on the dry sponge, would the sponge be soaking wet? The client will usually chuckle and respond with a resounding, "No." I will then illustrate that, over time, if we put one drop of water on the sponge over and over again, it will eventually soak it up and become supersaturated. I finish the analogy by saying that the more we do EMDR, the wetter their sponge will be. All in all, EMDR is an essential, empirically proven therapy that works wonders on trauma (Shapiro & Forrest, 1997).

So, what is it about one person that makes them able to handle a traumatic event where that same event will unhinge another person? When I began my journey into being a therapist, I talked to many firefighters. Some would say how the calls didn't bother them. I would hear this from one firefighter and then another would sidle up to me to bend my ear about the strife that they are going through. It seemed completely incongruent. With the fire service subscribing to a suck-it-up culture, it can be hard to find those who are suffering. I reflected on this. I worked with a hardened firefighter one time. Let's call him Jack. He was what we would call a firefighter's firefighter. This was always a compliment to the firefighter and their ability to carry on all the skills that were required of them – all while never forgetting where they came from if they were to climb up the promotional ladder. Jack was on an engine at the time as a firefighter/paramedic. His engine responded and rendered care for a patient until the ambulance could arrive. The call was for a nine year old girl who had just been raped. It wasn't even 10 o'clock. My partner and I arrived in the ambulance and met Jack and the patient. After making patient contact, we packaged the patient and released the engine company. Jack was adamant that he would go to the hospital since he had built rapport with her. I agreed. He was very compassionate, holding her hand and promising a peaceful outcome. After we dropped the patient off at the hospital, Jack returned to his engine and went back to quarters. Jack called me that night and asked for the patient's name so he could pray for her. I was a bit confused. In all the years I had known Jack, I had never seen him get emotional about a call, but this was the one that had affected him. "Jack," I asked him, "Why is this call different?" He responded without hesitation. "Her socks, Gregg. She had on Mickey Mouse socks just like my daughters."

So, I began researching what it was that allowed an event to affect one person but not the other. It wasn't until I participated in the Illinois Firefighter Peer Support Program (2021) that I learned about resiliency, which is, in its basic form, the ability to bounce back after adversity. They explained that there are both negative and positive effects of resiliency. The negatives included sleep deprivation, increased cortisol levels, and more. First, when we are sleep deprived, it increases our impulsive behavior. It also increases our emotional reactivity. Consider the young child who is up past their prescribed bedtime and how they are not emotionally regulated. In addition to this, when we are stressed, we produce more of the hormone Cortisol. When our body uses it appropriately, it regulates our blood pressure and sugar levels, but too much of this stress hormone will increase our blood pressure, make us fatigued, create medical problems such as headaches and stomach aches, and also increase our anxiety.

As I was taking this course, I began to get excited to know that there were things that people could do to improve their resiliency. These would be known as positive resilience factors.

When I looked at the list of these factors, I realized they were all very accessible to the average firefighter. The first one was to make connections. A good support system is paramount to having healthy resiliency. This includes having someone who is a positive influence on them, that they trust and who they can simply share their emotions with no matter the size of the issue. Or, they could be a part of a religious or civic organization that gives them access to help and support. Another positive factor was to be goal oriented or move towards a goal that is attainable. It doesn't have to be unreasonable, like being the general manager of a baseball team. It should be reachable, like trying to study hard for the Lieutenants exam or reading for pleasure more throughout the day. Taking decisive action seemed like an important positive factor to me. When faced with adversity, it is important to tackle it head on. So many of us bury our emotions or numb our sorrows in a glass of beer. The real work is done when we address our issues head on. The issues will not just up and vanish if we do not address them; they will eventually rear their ugly head in another form such as anxiety or depression. Finally, of course, there is the ability to care for ourselves. Exercise, take a walk, or spend time with family or friends. Whatever works for you. The goal is to care for yourself as much as you care for others on the job.

When I experienced major trauma, I felt like I was being punished. The sequence of events that unfolded thereafter were even more daunting as I tried to navigate the unknown. But it turned out it had more benefits than negatives. Sure, I suffered during this time. However, now I am able to empathize at the most profound level with my clients. Don't get me wrong, I would never wish trauma on anyone, but my experience with it has allowed me to connect in a way that is unimaginable.

ADJUSTING WELL

"I've got to admit it's getting better (better) a little better all the time (it can't get no worse)."

(Lennon & McCartney, 1967)

Picture it: you're having a bad day at work. The boss is on you every step, your deadlines are not being met, and your spouse is upset because you haven't been present for most of the week. You simply want to scream! What do you do to relieve stress? Many first responders will tell you that the best stress reliever is beer. Of course it is. When firefighters and paramedics get hired, it's to the bars they go. When someone at your firehouse gets promoted, let's have a party! Retirement? Suspension? Holidays? 4th of July? For cry-aye, St. Patrick's Day? It's all about the booze. The list goes on; however, this behavior, modeled by the senior members of our firehouses, promotes a lifestyle where bars become the liturgy of worship and drinking will heal all wounds.

I know that this chapter will be a bone of contention for many of the members of fire departments across America. The fire service is embedded in the culture of sharing a pint with their fellow firefighter. It is forever ingrained in the fabric that exists within the fire service. This is because it ignites the camaraderie that is so valuable to every firefighter whether old or new. Camaraderie is the hallmark of a healthy firehouse. It is found when dinner is done and everyone is cleaning up. The hustle and bustle of everyone is equal to the buzz found in a beehive. Everyone is doing their job. Meanwhile, there is banter that is exchanged. Joe makes fun of Tim for not washing his dish well enough before placing it in the dishwasher, Tim gloats about his rescue earlier that day, and Tanya is trying to take the credit because she is the one that placed the ladder Tim used to bring the child out of the window. How is this camaraderie created? Well, it starts when someone is a candidate.

When the academy is over and the firefighter is given a station assignment, they will come bearing gifts: a Danish, a box of doughnuts, some coffee. The items they bring will be judged and set the path of how the day will go. Throughout the next couple months, the candidate will be weighed, judged, evaluated, and more-basically, put through the ringer. He or she will do the dishes...*every day*. After some time, they will lead training to show their mastery. They will be ribbed, worked, made fun of, and if that wasn't enough, they still are not trusted until one thing happens...the first call where they can prove themselves to their fire company. After their first fire, if all goes accordingly, they will be welcomed into the fold of the firehouse. It is this rite of passage that allows them to be a part of the fire house. This is where camaraderie begins. It absolutely carries over when you are the detailed person at a house. You see, the regular crew at the firehouse have bonded over many calls. You are the outsider. Full stop. It is when, and only when, the rig has a legitimate call that requires others to work very hard – be it a fire or a pin-in accident, whatever the call may be – that the detailed person can speak freely and become forged into the firehouse lore.

Camaraderie is important. It is like having your tools ready to go. The hydraulic spreaders need to be tested, as do the saws. The engineer has to make sure the pump on the engine is functioning, and the others need to make sure the EMS equipment is accounted for. It is this potential energy that is important. It allows for us to spring into action and do our job well when called to do so. Conversely, it is the cohesiveness of the firehouse that allows them to function appropriately. If the housework is done efficiently and effectively, the officer does not have to worry about someone not doing what it is they are trained to do. My old Captain once told me that a really good shift comes along every once in a while and may last up to three years (until promotions and transfers will strip the shift apart). But, it is these shifts that make the officer feel like the king of the castle. When everyone is having fun coming back from a call, joking and laughing, it is then that the close-knit group has achieved their goal.

Friendships are made. Firefighters will get married, have children, and go through good times and bad. But it is these friendships that will allow them to go into battle with never a worry. So, when that call comes in and the pit of your stomach knows all too well that this address is a good address for a fire, it is then that the synergy of friendship is tested. When something goes awry, they will be there for you. When a shift has a bad call, it's to the bar they go to process the grief. I 100% agree with this process. It is essential in the growth of an individual or group to get over and process the issue they had. Be it a child that we could not resuscitate, or one of the fellas getting divorced, the bar with all my coworkers is where you would find me.

But, human behavior can dictate that this tradition may not be enough. Some may go with their friends, toss back a few, then go on to the side job like nothing has happened. Others may still have issues. You know when you eat popcorn and that one kernel gets stuck in your back molar, just out of reach for either your finger or your tongue? Grief is a lot like that. Like a little kernel, it persists, staying with you until you are forced to get a toothpick and pry it out of its temporary lair. Afterward, you sigh. For the popcorn kernel has been defeated!

Not everyone may find respite with the meeting of the crew. The grief may manifest in many other ways: anger, frustration, sadness, depression. Now, when this happens to someone, they may go to the firehouse the next shift and see everyone is okay. They all went out and had a beer. Everything was fixed. But, because *they* are not, they may not have the best way to deal with the emotions they are feeling. Anger could arise and to suppress it, John could go to the bottle of whiskey. Frustration could develop, and Tori will deal with her sorrows by starting a fight with her loved one. Ron will find out that his avoidance of his feelings will make it easy to have high-risk sexual relationships. Phil will not deal with things by enjoying the rush he gets when he gambles on football games. These, among other things, are what clinicians call maladaptive coping mechanisms. To break it down, when someone experiences negativity in their life, how they deal with the stimuli is an example of how they cope with something. When a person creates positive avenues in response to this stressor, it is considered an adaptive coping mechanism. These may include, but are not limited to, seeing a counselor, finding a way to physically deal with the stress (running, working out, playing sports), or meditation. The problem with firefighters is we are notorious for utilizing maladaptive coping mechanisms to deal with the nightmarish stressors we see on a daily basis. Stand-by for the tie-in…this is because of our culture within the fire service. Every milestone, every celebration, every time grief is dealt with, we turn to alcohol. It is so embedded in our culture that this is the go-to method for dealing with hard issues.

One of the techniques I use to show how bad maladaptive coping mechanisms, such as substance abuse, are is having the client make a T-Chart. On one side, we will write down the benefits of drinking. Typical answers include making them feel uninhibited, forgetting about the call, being happier, and enjoying sociability. Then, we will look at the negatives of drinking. Answers will usually be: possible criminal activity (drinking and driving), liver disease, reckless behavior like committing battery, and feeling ill the next day. I will then ask the client if they recognize a pattern between the two columns. Connecting the dots, we will surmise that the positives are short-term results and the negatives will reveal long-term consequences.

When looking at the growing body of research regarding Coping Theory, studies done by Lazarus and Folkman (1984) have been a mainstay since the mid 1980s. They explain that Coping Theory is when someone constantly changes their cognitive and behavioral efforts in order to manage internal and external demands. These demands are looked at as detrimental and too much for the person to handle. So, let's look at this for a minute. When an individual has a negative experience, say they were in a car accident, stress due to this can lead to the person feeling troubled and unprepared. They may be scared to get back into the car due to the risk of another accident happening. In order to combat these nerves, the person may try to do things that will combat this feeling. Doing so may be positive or negative, but the ultimate goal is to reduce the stress that has built up. This same person may cope in their own individualized way that they are comfortable with. Some may drink alcohol to help with the stress, while others may seek mental health counseling. Neither method is wrong or right, it is simply the way each person attempts to try to alleviate their stress. What makes it positive or negative is whether the person's mental well-being is increased or reduced.

When we look back, it is hard to ignore the father of modern psychology, Sigmund Freud, who taught about defense mechanisms. A defense mechanism is a psychological strategy that happens in our unconscious mind and is used to protect a person from having unacceptable thoughts or feelings (Cramer, 2000). These would be the predecessors to modern Coping Theory. We all know about the defense mechanism denial. This is when a person blocks external events from awareness. Another way to put it is, if someone was having problems dealing with a stimulus, they would simply not accept that it happened. An example of this is if a co-worker was relaying a story about you messing up at work – you might say that it never happened. This would be a classic example of denial. A defense mechanism that fascinates me is displacement. This is when you satisfy an impulse by substituting an object. If you are mad at your significant other, instead of releasing all hell on them, you may come home and yell at your dog that is not doing anything wrong. Defense mechanisms paved the way for other experts in the field to delve even deeper into a person's psyche, helping us to understand Coping Theory a bit better.

Building off of Freud's groundwork, Lazarus and Folkman's model (1984) created several examples of how successful coping mechanisms depend on emotional functions related to the problem. Simply put, when a large problem arises in our life, these are the ways that we might handle the issue:

Self-Control: how well we control our emotions when something stressful happens.

Confrontation: when a problem happens and we retaliate to make the problem benefit us.

Social Support: when we turn to our friends, acquaintances, and loved ones in order to help us during our time of need.

Emotional Distancing: when we prevent the problem from controlling what we do by remaining indifferent.

Escape and Avoidance: when we pretend that there is no stress at all.

Radical Acceptance: when the person is able to adapt to adversity by providing unconditional self-acceptance.

Positive Reappraisal: when the person grows by having the ability to find the answer in the struggle.

Strategic Problem-Solving: when the person uses solution-focused strategies in order to get through the tough time and move on.

Lazarus and Folkman (1984) continue to set the stage for us by explaining the difference between positive and maladaptive coping mechanisms. Remember, the coping mechanism is how we respond to the problem. By utilizing a more positive approach, we will come out the other end of the tragedy more well-adjusted and have fewer negative lingering effects. The first item they write about is having a good support system. There is nothing more powerful than to take the grief you are experiencing and share it with a confidant. The important takeaway is that your chosen person can be a loved one or simply someone that you trust and who can lend a listening ear to help you process the information. This could be a co-worker, someone else at the firehouse, or your significant other. If these two examples are not readily available, it may require you to step it up and find someone to talk to...a department

EAP is a great way to start. If anything, they can set you up for success by referring you to an appropriate level of care. By getting the issue that is spinning in your head to come out of your mouth, whether you know it or not, the healing has already begun. In addition to moving what ails you from your head space to your mouth space, the resource you are utilizing may provide positive feedback that might not be readily available to you in the mindset you are in.

If there is nobody readily available to discuss your issues, there are ways to properly cope with the adversity on your own. Relaxation is recommended in this scenario. As an aside, any positive coping mechanism can be used in conjunction with another. The benefits are compounded if this is utilized. So, the first thing you may ask is how you can even *think* about relaxing now that there is this horrible incident hanging around in your head. There is really no easy answer for this other than understanding that working on yourself is challenging. With this in mind, while the storm is volatile, it is extremely helpful to try and quell it. Ideally, this is done prior to the difficult incident occurring. If someone practices relaxation in their life, overcoming adversity can be optimized by utilizing your muscle memory. It is kind of like when a child is overstimulated. It is beneficial to calm them down in a way that is appropriate and aligned to their usual routine. The same works for us. One way to accomplish this is using mindfulness meditation. This is my favorite way to get people in touch with their inner calm. This is where the individual is talked to in a slow, relaxed, calm voice, placing them in a state of relaxation. Mindfulness meditation uses positive imagery to transport someone to a place of catharsis. I use mindfulness meditation in my practice regularly, and the reaction is always the same. Initially, the client feels weird because this may be out of their comfort zone. But at the end, they tell me how wonderful they feel, both in mind and body. The exciting thing about this is, with technology, mindfulness meditation apps are right at our fingertips. There are several apps that currently provide this, so a clinician isn't even needed to provide the service This allows the user to do it in their own safe space. The same result can be achieved through music. By listening to soothing music, the brain can reset and find a place of calm. The music provided for music therapy is often represented as waves, rainfall, animal sounds (such as whales, birds, etc.), and other ethereal sounds that will surely allow for a relaxed consciousness. Any of these techniques will support positive mental growth and allow the brain to relax. The more this is done, the better the muscle memory becomes. The brain can act like our muscles and, when a task is accomplished, it can bring you back to this time by using recall. Wouldn't you want your mind to be relaxed in a time of stress? I know I would.

I'm very lucky. Most of my clients are first responders. In order to make it in the fire service and be successful, it is imperative for the individual to be in great physical shape. When I went through the fire academy, I remember my drill instructor yelling at me as I dragged the weighted sled. "What sport were you in, Bagdade? Baseball? Football? Soccer?" my instructor shouted. "Nothing, Sir. I wasn't *in* sports," I replied, looking for a place to hide. He was searching for the words to respond. "Just use your legs, Bagdade!" Even though I did not play sports in high school, I understood the value of being physically fit. Physical wellness is a great way to properly cope with any stressor that may come your way. First off, anyone that has done physical activity knows the value of it afterward when the notorious endorphins (natural opiates found in the human body) release, leaving the person feeling great. This alone is a great way to stay motivated and continue to work on your physical wellness. Strength training, cycling and swimming can really boost someone's mood, allowing them to feel better both physically and mentally. But someone might ask, "What do I do if I am not into those things?" Yoga, stretching, or even brisk walks are activities that can be utilized to provide a low impact endorphin rush while maintaining positive physical health.

With every Yin, there must also be a Yang. Not everyone seeks out positive coping mechanisms. This could be because positive coping mechanisms take more energy to accomplish. Clinicians refer to when someone is affecting their wellbeing in a negative way as them having maladaptive coping mechanisms. These are much more accessible and take up less energy to accomplish. The first example of this is escape and avoidance. Much like Freud's example of denial, it is much easier for a person to rationalize that an incident simply did not happen than to deal with the hurt and the heartache that is associated with it. Firefighters are notorious for this. They may go on a call that involves much turmoil and they will simply push down the emotions so they do not have to deal with them. This is absolutely a survival technique and essential for first responders to get through their shift. Many of them work long hours. On CFD, we work 24 hour shifts. Within that time, we may see a multitude of different spectacles: someone shot by gunfire, a loved one passing away due to cancer, or pain and trauma suffered in an auto accident. The list goes on, inevitably. So, to go from call to call, these individuals will push down their emotions and earmark the incident so they can unpack it at a later time. Unfortunately, more often than not, they will never address the grief they experience. But, I assure you, the mind will remember. Pushing this down will result in the person having symptoms such as anger, depression, anxiety, and other fear-based issues that will occur at a later date. It is always important to eventually address these situations so your mental well-being can thrive and not be held back.

Many times when people are dealing with a stressor, they will do something that is familiar to them. When we resort to negative habits that are comforting to us, we call this dealing in the unhealthy comfort zone. What is more familiar to a firefighter than doing what it is we do more often than not? Yes, you got it! We will turn to drinking. Once again, for traditional camaraderie, having a pint with the guys and girls at your firehouse is perfectly acceptable. It becomes maladaptive when a couple things happen. If someone begins to drink by themselves, the practice becomes a bit more tedious. When I ask someone in session what the benefits of drinking are, they will notoriously say that it numbs them so they do not have to deal with the issue at hand. I would certainly take up a practice of ingesting a substance that makes all my heartache go away, right? Who wouldn't? But the bottom line is the consequences that supersede the benefits make this coping mechanism much less appetizing. In addition to alcohol, other unhealthy habits include drowning yourself in social media, eating excessively, or risky gambling. Anything that constitutes doing something unhealthy that someone would find is in their comfort zone would fall into this category.

If we are trapped within our own mind, with no way to express to others how we feel, a person may find themselves alone and without direction. Really, these are the situations that scare me the most. This is because when someone goes off the map, they may feel alone and isolated. When someone does this, they are trying to provide emotional numbing for themselves.

It matters not what the person does to cope with their situation. What does matter is that they are able to navigate the trauma in a healthy way that is comfortable for them. If someone has difficulty with the coping strategy, it is unlikely that they will revisit it. In counseling, we explore what works and what does not in order to achieve a more well balanced life for the client. The takeaway is that they will work on their mental health seriously and try to improve their present situation.

WORKING WITH A COUNSELOR

"I'm fixing a hole where the rain gets in, and stops my mind from wandering."
(Lennon & McCartney, 1967)

When I started my Bachelor's program at Penn State, I was well aware that I would have difficulty in the whole process of going back to school. Finding time to write papers, studying terms on notecards, this jaunt back to academia was enough to keep a large supply of Excedrin Migraine on hand, for sure! I remember during my first semester my wife told me to take classes that I would enjoy. So, I signed up for Humans as Primates because I always had an affinity for animals and the fossil record. When the class was completed, I ran to the nearest computer to reveal my impending score. Being a C+ student my whole scholastic career, I was expecting to follow suit in my old ways. A few keystrokes later and... *all A's?!* My brain could barely comprehend the information my eyes were filtering in. Kismet has a way of messing with an individual. For example, when someone goes to Las Vegas for the first time, their beginner's luck will surely net them a glorious bounty, steering them into a large amount of confidence from there forward. I was *not* going to be fooled by the likes of these antics. Next semester, all A's and one B! The subsequent semesters seemed to follow suit in this similar trajectory. I was on a roll, until I had to take *Algebra*. I shudder writing that word to this very day. Math was my weak point, my Achilles heel, my nemesis. I grabbed all the confidence I could by mustering up what I had accomplished during the last multiple semesters and took the placement exam. The results read something like this:

Mr. Bagdade,

It has come to our attention that you have recently completed the Math placement exam. After reviewing the results, we have determined that you are not qualified for anything that involves any type of math expression, whatsoever. We can offer you a remedial class in Algebra as a consolation; however, it will be expensive and will not count toward your degree audit. Please consider giving up, as it is an easier alternative to the hell you will face ahead of you.

Signed,

The Entire Math Department.

I ended up taking the remedial course and aced it. The final straw was ahead of me. The College Algebra course at Penn State was like a really good hockey game. There were ups; there were downs. When all hope was exhausted, a shining light of victory would appear. I hired a tutor for the final who turned out to be a large Ukrainian man who would yell at me until I got the answer correct. After the final, I went to my computer. I pressed the keys with one hand while shielding my eyes with the fingers on my other hand. And the final grade was...

C-. C-! I jumped for joy. C-! I had passed College Algebra, and this would be the only class I would get less than a B in my whole collegiate career. Now, all I have to do is get past Statistics and everything would be hunky dory.

My understanding of math is that some people comprehend Algebra better than Geometry, or vice versa. It just makes more sense to them. If you ask anyone who has attended college, they will tell you that Statistics is one of the worst courses they have taken. I returned to my computer and, with great dread, enrolled in the course. But, my wife nicely placed the power of suggestion on me for this situation. She simply said to me that Statistics is an essential part of my would-be career and that I should embrace this course. "Who knows? You might enjoy it!" She quipped. I not only aced it, but my wife was right. It was strangely enjoyable.

One of the exciting things about Statistics is the idea that with research, a study can prove something more worthy than another. For example, as I entered my career as a counselor, I found there were copious amounts of theories, techniques, and models that I could use in my practice. What would distinguish one from another would be if it had been tested. It is the scientific way to take an idea that was thought of one way and expound on it in a different light. I promised to myself that I would do work that was empirically tested and thoroughly vetted by a multitude of people that are a lot smarter than me so my clients would have the optimum care ahead of them.

Techniques that I use quite often come from the world of EMDR, but have roots in Dialectical Behavioural Therapy (DBT). Some call them grounding techniques, others may refer to them as mindfulness. Ultimately, the goal is the same and the client will arrive at a more present, less anxious place. When someone is suffering from emotional trauma, they may reveal this in many ways. The client can reveal to you, the clinician, that they are simply angry, or they may tell you that they have thoughts that they cannot control. Another might tell you that they have copious amounts of anxiety that cripple them in some situations. Any way it is packaged, the symptom is a summation of its parts. There is trauma that is causing this notion. There are some techniques that must be done with another person, and there are others that the client can do individually. Both are appropriate, however, the client will sometimes rely on the counselor for this additional help, so the techniques they can do on their own would prove to be quite useful. The goal is to allow the client to become completely present. When the anxiety, anger, ruminating thoughts, or whatever ails them starts, it is mostly in the client's head. They are, essentially, suffering from a state that, much like a feedback loop, does not allow them to recognize the outside world. In order to combat this, it is essential to get them to not only recognize that there is a whole world right in front of their nose, but that they can become calm by doing simple techniques.

When someone is feeling this way, they can do something comparable to the explanation of combing one's hair. Picture it. You have come home from a horrible day at work. The stress of the day is eating you alive and now you must come home to two rowdy children and a demanding spouse. As you digest this, the anxiety fills your whole being almost to the point of not being able to function. Mindfulness allows us to focus our energy on the here and now, bringing us back to reality and taking us out of our head. This can be done by combing one's hair. Now, it would be safe to assume that the subject has hair prior to this explanation, but some (like myself) are folliclely challenged. But, the notion fits many bills and can be rebranded in many different ways. When the client takes the hairbrush in their hand, and they slowly brush their hair in a methodical way, they are now focusing their attention outwardly. They are feeling the handle of the brush, they are feeling their hair run through the teeth of the brush, and their scalp has a sensation all its own. Whatever was going on in the client's head has now been absorbed by the efforts of combing their head. This process forces them to become present and aware of where they are in the world, right now. No longer will they be thinking about all the ills prior to the combing of the hair.

A common technique that is used to achieve this is commonly called the Five Senses Technique. The counselor asks the client to gather in their surroundings. The client will then look around and recite five things that they see in their field of vision. Next, the counselor will ask the client to tell them four things they can hear. After their response, the counselor will follow up by asking the client for three things they can touch, two things they can smell, and one thing they can taste. The client is allowing themselves to be present in their life and will no longer be stuck in their head space. With existing trauma, the fight/flight/freeze response is overcome by doing this simple exercise. The client's anxiety level will come down to a manageable level.

Some techniques can be done by the individual themselves. These are desirable when the client is not with the counselor and would like to represent mindfulness by themselves. My daughter and I have played a game for many years that I feel is a useful tool in my practice when I have a client that presents with anxiety, anger, ruminating thoughts, or any other trauma related behavior. This is called the Rainbow Technique. When the client's symptoms come on, they can find something in their environment that is representative of the colors of the rainbow. Red, orange, yellow, green, blue, purple. My daughter and I would be driving along and spot cars on the road that are representative of these colors. We would be careful to find them in the order that they are presented in the rainbow itself, but once this was exhausted, we would do the reverse of the original plan. Purple, blue, green, yellow, orange, and red. This can be done as many times as required to allow the client to become present and overcome whatever it is that is ailing them at the time. The client can also measure their anxiety prior to the exercise (on a 1-10 scale), as well as after the exercise in order to see if they have improved.

The mind is quite complex. However, at times, it can hinder our growth. These techniques, in addition to many other items that can allow the client to become present, are useful in many ways. Much of talk therapy is deciphering what it is the client is experiencing and finding a way to combat the unnecessary behavior. Working with a counselor will allow the client to find ways that work for them specifically. It is common knowledge that what might work for me, might not work for you. The difference between a good counselor and a great counselor (aside from rapport) is marked improvement of the client. I oftentimes ask clients that have been in therapy for a long time what they expect now that is different from past experiences with counseling. Because isn't it the goal for the client to have resolve from their main issues? I would like to think so. When someone goes to an orthopedist for tendonitis of the knee, it is the goal of the specialist to resolve the client's pain and return them to a path of full functioning. The same goes for treating mental health.

Now, relatively speaking, every counselor is not suited for every client. Some clients prefer same sex counselors. Others prefer counselors of the opposite sex. One of the most valuable items when picking a suitable counselor is using a little research. First, every counselor has their target population they want to work with. For example, some counselors prefer to treat children. Others like working with addiction. Sometimes, the population a counselor works with correlates with the adversity they may have dealt with in their personal life. The takeaway is that counselors prefer to work with certain populations. Finding someone that fits your issues takes a little bit of research, but can go a long way. Many professional databases will provide this information when reaching out to a counselor.

Once the appropriate counselor has been chosen from the pool, the plight is not over. A good counselor will spend the first couple sessions trying to develop rapport with the client. Finding common ground is essential to allowing the counselor into your world. If a child is into collecting Pokémon cards, it would behoove the counselor to talk about this with the client. When the client is in an environment where they are sharing parts of their world that they enjoy, I wholeheartedly assure you the counselor will benefit. My situation is not like others. I am a firefighter and a counselor. This has placed me in an environment that makes me uniquely qualified to treat firefighters because I have been in many situations throughout my career that allow me to empathize with my clients. It goes hand-in-hand with why firefighters often couple with nurses and police officers. At the end of the day, it is easier to explain to them the main story, instead of explaining the job specific details. My clients often tell me that they like coming to me because they can tell me a story about work and I will be able to relate to them sincerely. Now, I would be a fool if I told you that you had to go to a counselor that is/was a firefighter. We simply are not that prevalent. So, what are you supposed to do? It comes down to how well you work with the counselor and how much preparation they have had on the subject you are in need of.

There are a growing number of counselors that care for first responders. Some are, or were, in the fire service; others have a spouse or family member that is a firefighter. Others are just interested in working with this population and specialize in the psychological needs of a firefighter. One of the most common misnomers I hear from firefighters is they do not understand the differences between each of the specific mental health professionals that they would go and see. Allow me to explain this. A *Psychiatrist* is a doctor and has been through medical school. This is the highest level in the profession. Their aim is to assess, diagnose, and prescribe various psychotropic medications to their clients and evaluate them regularly. Next is the *Psychologist*. Psychologists have schooling that takes them through to the Doctoral level, which makes them doctors, but not medical doctors. In the clinical setting, they can administer various complex assessments and do talk therapy. They cannot administer medication to their clients. *Social Workers* and *Professional Counselors* are Master's level clinicians. Their aim is to provide talk therapy from a holistic means, drawing from a multitude of theories and models. My personal and professional opinion is, whether educated to the Doctoral level or Master's level, a qualified, professional, appropriate therapist is worth their weight in gold. Moving to a higher level of education is not necessary, unless that clinician is well versed in the requirements that the individual needs. Ultimately, it comes down to comfort level, knowledge, and rapport. During the first couple sessions, it is your responsibility to ask questions of your therapist that you require answers to. The street goes both ways. If it's not working for you, do not feel abashed about canceling the helping relationship and finding a better fit. Being your own advocate and knowing what is good for you is essential to your own personal growth.

TAKE CARE OF MYSELF? WHY?

"With every mistake we must surely be learning."
(Harrison, 1968)

Growing up in the suburbs of Chicago, I lived a very stereotypical childhood. Whether fishing at the local watering hole, playing whiffle ball with my friends after school, or running around the neighborhood at night playing Ghost in the Graveyard, I found catharsis in the everyday. Pick up games of football and baseball not only cemented friendships, but taught us that autonomy was a good thing. Our parents trusted us. They allowed us to go into the neighborhood after school and all summer long, etching these moments into our memories long after childhood. My father would regularly take my brother and I to the forest preserve. We would walk around the woods picking up pine cones and listening to the cicadas' melody as they swooned their mates. I always loved the smell of the earth. The forest, to me, was an allegory to the life cycle. Within the rich, lustrous ground were seeds shed by large oak trees. These seeds yield life, growing from a fragile sapling into a large, unwavering tree. After years of growth, the inevitable will happen. The oak tree will lay down and provide nutrients for a plethora of living things, creating life once again. The forest provided a meditative arena for my chaotic mind to rest. I could put aside the overstimulation of life and simply be.

With all of the wonderful things my childhood provided, I would soon find out that adversity is really what shapes an individual. At the tender age of seven, I started blinking and jerking my head uncontrollably. Doctors at the time couldn't pinpoint what the issue was. After a lot of medical experimentation, the doctors finally had something to say, "Your son has Tourette's Syndrome." My mother and father replied, "Is he going to die?" When they found out that it was non-fatal, the next step was to make me stick out less than an infected toe. Unfortunately, this was not accomplished. At 7 years old, my parents made me stand up in front of my whole class and "educate them" on why I was so different. Talk about social suicide! I remember showing them the reel-to-reel of a movie called, *Stop it, I can't* (Williams, 2014).

An informative, yet dated, educational film on the ins and outs of Tourette's Syndrome. The purpose was to educate. I do look back at these events and see that my parents were actually doing everything they could with the toolbox they had. But, the years that unfolded were filled with isolation, self-loathing, and desperation.

When I got to high school, I surrounded myself with people who did drugs. It provided me with an escape from my loneliness, and I felt like I deserved nothing better than the damage I would do to my mind, body, and soul. As an aside, I did also discover music, and I believe that is what drives me to this very day (in nothing but the most positive way). There was never a time where I wanted to hurt myself, but I know in my heart of hearts that I was very mad at myself. I did not like who I was. I mention this not as a caution to others, but more of a point of self-reflection. I do believe that to arrive at destination C, you must first live through A and B. I remember an episode of a cartoon I liked to watch as a child called, *Thundercats*. There was one particular episode where Lion-o, the main character, had to go through a series of tests that involved strength, dexterity, and cognition. Lion-o needed to accomplish each of these challenges in order to arrive on the other side, better than he was before (Rankin/Bass Animated Entertainment, 1985-1988). After pontificating the summation of these parts, I believe that we become who we are because of what we go through in our younger years.

As life ticks on, we find more and more reason to create a conglomerate of busy work. This could be masked as someone burying their life in their work. Many couples have separated because of this idea. The story is as old as the human race. Take Jane for example. Jane works to find people mortgages for their newly purchased homes. She was promised a 40-hour work schedule when she first got hired. But, as time went on, she found herself coming to work early and burning the midnight oil to get ahead of the game. Of course, she masked this process by saying she wanted to make a good impression on the company. This soon turned into more hours, more paperwork, and less time for Jane. After three years of establishing herself with her colleagues, Jane felt like she no longer had a life; or rather, her work *was* her life. She stopped going out with her friends. Dating was no longer an option since Jane had deadlines to reach. This certainly could not be interrupted. If we peel back the layers of Jane's life, we can actually see the real reason she fell into this behavior is because she was stuck in a feedback loop that she was not able to get out of.

"I'll take Unreasonable Behavior for 1000 points, Alex."

"The answer is: This is the reason why Jane craves work more than anything else in her life…Gregg?"

"What is *control*?"

Yes, Jane feels most in control of her life when she sits down at her desk, speaks with the spanking new homeowner, and applies her knowledge to get them the loan they so desperately need. This control allows her to sacrifice her own happiness. Period.

First responders are notorious for this behavior. It usually starts with the hiring process. When we begin our career, we must jump through many hoops in order to land the coveted dream job. There is physical preparation. We must be in tip top shape in order to pass very competitive physical fitness standards. We must be scholastically capable. There is usually a written examination that must be completed, and only the highest scores will move on to the next round. There is an oral interview. We must be poised and professional, wowing the officers with our charisma in the hopes that we will go on to the next level. All of these steps require hours of preparation. And so it begins. The dream job that so many of us worked so hard to land. "Hey! Wanna get promoted? You gotta take Fire Officer I!" "Wanna go to a busier spot? You really should take RIT Under Fire and Trench Rescue." The list goes on and on as our career unfolds.

Overtime is a carrot that most are willing to take because of the reward. But is it really worth it? Our Paramedics in the city work on a four-platoon system. They work a 24-hour shift and they are off for 72-hours. If they get an overtime shift, they will work on their mirror shift. So, if they are on the first shift normally, they will be off for second shift, third shift and fourth shift. Sounds great, right? But, when the overtime carrot dangles, they work 24 hours on first shift, off on second shift, work 24 hours on third shift, off on fourth shift. Then lo and behold, their normal shift is back again! 24 hours *on*. 24 hours *off*. 24 hours *on*. 24 hours *off*. 24 hours *on*. Make no mistake – this is blood money, people! The lack of quality sleep *alone* will put someone in a tizzy!

So, what can we do to combat this? There has got to be a way to take care of one's self while living up to the obligation they promised to their employer. In counseling, we refer to this as Work/Life Balance. When someone is in my office, I give them a piece of paper and a pen, and I have them draw a circle. I tell them that the circle is the whole of how they spend their life. I then tell them to divide up the circle into different parts: Social, Sleep, Work, Hobbies, Family, etc. They must measure out how much each of these constructs is accomplished with a larger pie wedge or smaller. People are often dumbfounded at what they put! The second part of this is to complete the exercise again: once when they begin therapy and another after months of therapy. Usually, the pie chart changes for the better.

One of the first concepts I introduce to clients is a concept I refer to as *a moment of catharsis*. The way I describe it to them is like so:

I own a Jeep Wrangler. I have a playlist of songs that I like to play when the top of my Jeep is down, convertible style. As I am driving along, the sun hits my face on this bright sunny day. I smell the trees as I drive by them. The song *Mr. Blue Sky* by Electric Light Orchestra comes on and I am feeling very good at this moment. As a matter of fact, I feel *great*! It is at this moment that I am most content. I am having a moment of catharsis.

I will work with clients to find ways to tap into this meditative state. It certainly is a healthy exercise in caring for one's mental health in a positive way, while being present (which is always a good thing). My hope is for others to find their own moment of catharsis however it manifests in their own life, with stimuli that create an atmosphere much like the one I portrayed. I will then have them use this moment as a positive template when things are going awry for them. Oftentimes, first responders may feel anxious due to the call volume. I would instruct them to try and tap into this template by allowing themselves to feel wondrous and less weighted down. I would say to think of a moment where you are happy, relaxed, and without worry. They would follow suit by describing their moment of catharsis. By meditating on this, it will help place them in a state of relaxation, and hopefully they will have less of a cortisol rush (a stress hormone) and more of an endorphin rush (a pleasure hormone).

When I was a young paramedic, I learned about heart disease. My understanding of it was that there are controllable as well as uncontrollable factors that can affect our susceptibility to having atherosclerosis (or hardening of the arteries as it is commonly known). Uncontrollable factors would be genetics, age, and gender. Studies have proven that if you are over 50, male, and have a family history of heart disease, then there is a real chance that you will develop it as well. The controllable factors were much more interesting to me. Some of these are smoking status, what comprises your diet, how often you exercise, and monitoring your cholesterol/blood pressure. I was dumbfounded to discover this information. You mean to tell me that I am in *control* of whether or not I have heart disease? My childhood mentor, Yoda from the Star Wars

Trilogy, would certainly weigh in on this. "Do, or do not. There is no try!" (Lucas, 1977). It is important to empower yourself to follow suit and be in charge of your destiny.

This concept directly translates to self-care for the first responder. Self-care is the controllable variable that we can use to be at one with ourselves and the universe. Firefighters know this concept well. When a house is on fire, the superheated gasses make firefighting extremely intense due to churning smoke conditions and unbearable heat. The longer the house burns, the worse this phenomenon proliferates. An intervention is needed to stop this. According to standard operating procedures, a truck company will place a ventilation hole in the roof, allowing the gas, smoke, and fire to escape and making a clear path for the engine company to extinguish the seat of the fire. This can be likened to a tea kettle that, when the water begins to boil, lets out a whistle to allow for the pressure to be released.

People experience this during everyday affairs. Between work, family life, social responsibilities, and dedication to clubs and organizations, an individual may feel overwhelmed. The constraints they feel are real and may show up in their life in a negative manner. They may feel overwhelmed, stressed, overworked, and anxious. Enter our controllable friend *self-care*! There are things that one can do on a daily basis that can prevent their tea kettle from building too much pressure. There are many models of self-care, but they all contain four main dimensions: Physical, emotional, psychological, or spiritual. First, there is the physical dimension. In addition to eating healthy and drinking lots of water, it is important to treat your body as if it is a temple. Wait! I've heard that before! By caring for it with regular exercise, moments to rest, and a regular massage, your body will thank you by feeling good both inside and out. Next, is looking at the dimension defined for the psychological mind. Our mind is thirsty for knowledge. That is the reason we need constant stimulation. Cultivating this dimension is important for maintaining your brain power. What works for you may not work for others, so it is important to be introspective and find what works for you, specifically. Some psychological self-care examples include reading a good book or magazine. If you are a gamer, it might mean playing chess or cards. Many people find it important to do meditation or have a cerebral conversation with a close friend. Emotional self-care is important as well. Setting appropriate boundaries is super important within this dimension. If you can allow others to love you unconditionally, then loving yourself follows suit. By doing this, you will become more self-aware, allowing for true self-love. This dimension allows for you to be inspired. Friends and family activities, a love of animals, and charitable work will allow for this to be fulfilled. Finally, the spiritual dimension (to me) is the most important. This is a great time to use prayer or meditation to get in touch with identifying what is meaningful to you. Two important ideas for this dimension could be being one with nature and practicing gratitude. Walking in a forest preserve or taking your dog to the dog park may help you attune with something much larger than yourself. The most important takeaway from this is, some examples might not work for others. Creating a self-care plan that works for *you* will not only make you want to follow it, but will release the much needed stress that tends to build up regularly in your life (Taylor, et.al., 2011).

HOW CAN I HELP?

"Help me if you can, I'm feeling down and I do appreciate you being 'round. Help me get my feet back on the ground. Won't you please, please help me?"

(Lennon & McCartney, 1965)

Prior to getting my Master's degree in counseling, I had to get my Bachelor's degree. I was blessed that I could go back to school by doing the whole program online. Throughout high school, I was a B/C student. I remember telling my mother that there was nothing wrong with getting a C in a class because it was an *average* mark. "Mom! There is nothing wrong with being average!" My mother would try to instill in me that I was not only above average, but I was *remarkable*. At that time, I simply did not believe this. So, average is where I found my place.

My parents were more supportive than most parents. I remember coming home from school and presenting a project that I had worked on to them. They would beam with joy, telling me that it would surely be placed in a museum next to Picasso's works of art. If anyone has seen the sitcom *The Goldbergs*, I would swear on a stack of Beatles records that my mother went to a parental camp with the mother on that tv show (Goldberg, et.al., 2022). But the rest of our relationship was open and full of life lessons. I was able to process life's ills with them, constantly evaluating what I did right and what I did wrong.

College, while working and having a family, was no joke. I remember coming back from running a call on Engine 113 and trying to write an eight page paper on climate change. The semester I took Greek and Roman Mythology was reading intensive. I was *literally* reading 24/7 during this class! I remember reading Homer, Ovid, and all the regulars that made up this genre, in record time. One of the stories that stuck out was the story of Sisyphus. Sisyphus was punished by the gods and was ordered to serve the rest of his life rolling a boulder up a hill, only to have it roll down to him again. This feedback loop is synonymous with the plight many people have when they suffer from mental illness. They feel like life is futile, much like the perpetual futility of the work Sisyphus had to endure.

My Lieutenant at the time would often ask me what I wanted to be when I grew up. We shared a good laugh, since I was deep into my fire service career and here I was, an adult college student, trying to obtain higher education. He would say, "I'm at the *end* of my career and I still don't know what I want to do!" I replied that he'll eventually figure it out and we both had a chuckle. Since online learning was relatively new at this time, my coworkers would equate it with an easier, non-comprehensive degree. The big online degree during this time was University of Phoenix, and while there was nothing wrong with this school, my co-workers worked hard to poke fun at its legitimacy. They would habitually mock my schooling by pretending to flap their wings, cawing like a crow. "You're a phoenix, Gregg! Rise from the ashes!" Now this would faze most people since it is important to gain the favor of our co-workers, especially at my own firehouse. But I heard what they were actually saying loud and clear. They were saying they were proud of me, and that they couldn't fathom putting in the work that I was. Firefighters compliment others in a very backhanded way. It's not meant to be hurtful; it's just how we operate. For example, if someone did a wonderful job on the ambulance, saving someone's life or performing a valiant rescue on the fireground, their peers would certainly bust their stones relentlessly by referring to them as the hero who must be addressed accordingly. This was definitely not the showering of praise that Mom and Dad Bagdade gave me throughout the years! It's okay. It builds character while making sure that it doesn't go to your head. It may not be well understood by the general public, but firefighters perform lifesaving acts every day. Yes, when someone experiences a traumatic event or a serious illness that is meant to take their lives, it is these wonderful men and women who step in and challenge destiny with their knowledge of lifesaving procedures, as well as their aggressive ability to adapt to conditions that are unbelievably challenging. When you go to work and know that multiple times throughout the day, you may provide a lifesaving intervention, it is easy for it to go to your head and inflate your ego. The playful ribbing that our co-workers provide is not only important to keep someone's ego in check, it is present to develop the ongoing camaraderie that we cherish so much.

Prior to graduating from this program, I needed to secure an internship. I approached the director of the Human Relations Department of the Chicago Fire Department to see if I could participate in the Employee Assistance Program. After all, what better way to see if I could help my fellow co-workers than to be placed in a position where I could do exactly that? I was accepted and spent two semesters in that capacity. One of my first responsibilities was to be the liaison for the new Social Worker that was hired. I would be the catalyst for her to enter the firehouses, introducing her to the rank and file and normalizing the importance of mental health within the fire service. I learned much in this capacity. I was able to help my co-workers in a new and exciting way. One thing that I learned during this time was a valuable lesson. When people would come down to the EAP office to get help with their situation, the director of the program would ask them if they'd like to talk to me. One of two scenarios would come into play. They would either say, "Gregg? I'd *love* to talk to him, he gets it!" *or,* "Gregg? I can't talk to Gregg...I know him too well." The former response would make me feel worthy and informed. I *did* get it, being a peer that stood side by side on calls with many of them. The latter response was just as important to me. It showed me that the familiarity people had with me was a deterrent to getting help. It wasn't because of my knowledge of the subject at all; it was because they knew me and might have issues divulging information for fear of a possible breach of privacy.

I learned two valuable lessons regarding this. First, it would be important for me to stress confidentiality while seeing these people as my future clients. Maintaining this would allow them to relax and feel confidence that their information will not spill into the firehouse where others may know their situation. Counselors know that rapport is key in order to get to the bottom of what ails the individual. If there is no confidentiality, then the clinician can basically kiss the rapport out the window. I pride myself now in that my practice is a half hour drive out of the city of Chicago, forcing those that come see me from the city to take multiple expressways to get to my office. This space allows for a physical representation of what confidentiality looks like. Indeed, I maintain confidentiality as well. I would not have buy-in from my clients if I did not. Confidentiality stands as a pillar in my practice.

The other aspect of me knowing the client too intimately had me thinking, too. I *did* understand what they were going through and could probably provide insight that others might not be able to pinpoint, but what is the use if the client is not comfortable sharing their situation with me? To this I say that the most important factor at play here is that the client seeks help regardless of who it is, as long as they do seek the help they need. When I speak to new clients, especially those within the fire service, I assure them of two things: I will remain 100% confidential and if I cannot help you, I will make it a point to find someone who can. At my practice, we have clinicians that are well qualified to treat most mental health situations. I provide supervision for these clinicians to ensure that they understand the world of the fire service, since it is such a niche subculture.

During this undergraduate internship, I was asked to join the CFD Peer Support Program. A program like this is essential to the positive mental health of its members. Realistically, the role of the peer supporter is to be activated when a member of the fire department has had a traumatic call that may overwhelm them afterward. It is the goal of the peer supporter to assess the member's overall well-being and provide comfort in their time of need. The peer supporter is simply a tourniquet on an arterial wound. They are there to stop the proverbial bleed. During my time as a peer supporter, I would respond to firehouses, voluntarily, for various emergencies. My first goal was to allow the first responder to gain my trust. I was no longer Gregg the Firefighter. I was Gregg the Peer Supporter. This was a different hat to wear. Even in these instances, rapport was vital; it provided an opening into what most would like to not uncover. But, unlike individual therapy, a peer supporter is not there to solve any problems. They are simply there to listen. By listening to the member's ills, it gets the horrible incident from their head space to their mouth space. Just getting it out of their head provides the first step in the healing process. The next step is to validate their emotions. What this means is the peer supporter must make it okay for the member to feel what they are feeling. If they are mad about the call, let them be mad. If they are devastated about the results, let them be devastated. This validation of emotion allows the member to know that what they are feeling is not only normal, but okay and allowed. The next step is to provide sympathy or empathy. Not everyone knows the difference between the two, but it is actually quite simple. Sympathy is when *you* experience something and I haven't. I can be there for you the best I can, but I don't know exactly what you've been through. Empathy is when I have had a similar experience as *you*. I can understand with every fiber of my body what you are going through. Not only can I be there for you, but I understand what it is that is affecting you, because I was there, too. The final caveat for peer support is you are not there to fix the issue. Period. You are there to be there for the member and allow them to vent. Any solutions should be heeded, and it is not the peer supporter's responsibility. If the peer supporter has done a good job, the affected member should feel supported and comforted and they should have a measurable difference in negative emotion.

A couple years ago, I went to a symposium put on by the Illinois Firefighter Peer Support organization (2021). They are a conglomerate of firefighters and clinicians who have banded together to provide a service in educating departments about peer support programs, as well as providing a network of clinicians that can help members if they are in need. The symposium was not only a great way to network, it was a bevy of information, with representatives from all over the spectrum with one goal in mind…to put firefighter mental health at the forefront of people's minds. I walked around, made some connections, watched some presenters, and came out feeling inspired. The director of the symposium gave his introductory speech, and it was awe-inspiring.(Illinois Firefighter Peer Support, 2021). He shared a story of a river. This river was unique. It had been troublesome for some time. You see, it was the life source for the village nearby. But what brings life, may also bring death. Villagers would come to the banks and get the water they so desperately needed. However, something was amiss. People were falling into the river in record numbers. The villagers were exhausted from chasing the fallen down the river to save them from its wrath. After much time, someone would fall in the river and the villagers would continue to do the same: run down the river and rescue them from certain death. One day, the village elder said, "Why do we run down the river to rescue the villagers who have fallen in?" Dumbfounded, the chorus responded with disdain, "Because if we do not, they will surely die!" The village elder was quick to respond, "Ah, but what would it look like if we went upstream and found the reason why the villagers are falling in? What if we could fix that?" (2021).

This story is a prime example of why it is important to be *proactive* with mental health within the fire service. When we are *reactive*, it is already too late, and we are behind the eight ball.

That is why it is vital to be on top of firefighter mental health. The State of Illinois has required a minimum amount of education to be spent on talking about such things as anxiety, depression, signs of someone that is suffering from a mental health crisis, and more during fire service training. By normalizing this training, fire service personnel will be more inclined to find out the why of mental health, and simply normalizing it will set up the next generation of firefighters for success.

Early in my career, I learned the answer to this question: what is the first thing you do when responding to a fire? Most will answer that they will assess the building from three sides and plan accordingly. But what would it look like if you had been to this building prior to this fire? What if you had looked around it and determined the most prudent way to attack a fire that may happen there? Where to place the ladders, where the fire hydrants were located. This pre-planning would be essential and provide insight for the responding firefighters, as they had first-hand knowledge of this building prior to the conflagration ahead of them. Ultimately, it is this same mode of thinking that must envelop mental health training within the fire service.

When a crisis has occurred on the fire ground, it is imperative to make sure the people that are helping others get the help they need. It is easy to assume that firefighters are invincible, but the reality is that they have thoughts and feelings just like everyone else. When a traumatic event occurs at work, a counselor will provide a service called Critical Incident Stress Debriefing (CISD). This is a multilevel program that involves having firefighters share what they saw on the scene of the troubling incident, learning awareness regarding future reactions and having access to resources, if needed. Traditionally, the debriefing happens shortly after the incident, within 72 hours. When a CISD is issued, it is usually headed by a licensed therapist who will have all of the firefighters sit at a table together and begin working on the incident. Although I understand the necessity of this process, I feel the program is flawed in many ways. First off, when an incident happens (it matters not if the fire department is small or large) the personnel are in disarray. At times, manpower must be shuffled, stress levels are at an all time high, and the *last* thing the crew wants to do is talk about how they feel in front of their comrades. In theory the program is optimum, but in the world of the fire service, it may not be practical. First, it may be challenging for firefighters to discuss the incident without judging each other. It is in our nature to Monday morning quarterback every incident. This means that others will review the incident and respond with how it should have gone another way. During this trying and emotional time, it is essential that people's emotions be met with compassion and not criticism. This type of criticism should be held in a different forum such as an After Incident Critique. Another roadblock for a traditional CISD is it might be hard for firefighters to express emotion in front of their peers as it might be viewed as weakness. Due to the competitive nature of our job, we are conditioned to be the best *at all times*, regardless of adversity (Mitchell & Everly, 1997).

I feel there should be a better way to approach a critical incident. For example, what if instead of one therapist discussing the incident with a whole group of firefighters, there were multiple therapists that visited the firehouse. They could reach out to the firefighters in their own way. Not everyone handles large amounts of stress the same way. Some of us can't tell enough people how we are feeling, while others may have trouble talking about the incident and just keep it to themselves. Our way of handling stress is different as well. One person may become very emotional and cry a lot. Others may revert to their bunk and isolate themselves. The therapists could discuss the incident with those involved in their own chosen environment. If someone is in their bunk, then that might be where the incident is discussed. If a couple members are shooting hoops or throwing a ball around, it is here that the therapist will have to set up shop. In the counseling community it is called meeting the client where they're at. By doing this, firefighters are more willing to share what they are feeling with the therapist. It makes them more accessible to a reclusive group that is not used to receiving this kind of help.

The ultimate goal is to be proactive and find ways to help firefighters with their mental health. Whether it be an officer who assesses their crew daily, or someone starting up a peer support team within their department, the goal is to be available for this population. If we cannot help those that protect the home front, then who will protect us?

MARRIAGE, FAMILY, AND PETS

"When I find myself in times of trouble, Mother Mary comes to me, speaking words of wisdom, let it be. And in my hour of darkness, she is standing right in front of me speaking words of wisdom, let it be."
(Lennon & McCartney, 1970)

When I was single, there was always a draw to my profession from potential romantic partners. Be it the uniform, the nature of the profession, or the cliché of a rugged firefighter helping someone in need, there was no shortage of people that were interested. I blame the media and those ridiculous calendars! But, I digress. Realistically, once the shininess wears off, the realities of the profession will certainly rear their ugly heads. I mean who really wants a sleep-deprived, adrenaline junkie that is sure to be on shift when all things at home go to pot? I assure you, when the hot water heater decides it no longer wants to work, or Junior gets hit with a rock, requiring several stitches to his chin, it will indubitably be your significant other that will be required to pick up the slack.

When I graduated from the fire academy (the second time around – this time becoming a firefighter), I was married with children. My son was two and a half years old and my daughter was six months old. The ceremony was held at Navy Pier's Grand Ballroom in Downtown Chicago. It was quite an extravagant affair. All of us firefighters were squared away in our dress blues, carefully practicing our marching into the facility and feeling on top of the world. The ceremony was just about to start. We were feeling confident and prepared. I peeled back the curtain and gazed into the audience. There was no sign of my wife and kids! I excused myself and made a quick phone call to her. I asked, "Where *are* you? We are about to go on any minute!" If I only knew the treachery that she had been through, I would have thought twice about placing that call. I would find out the story later on that night. In brief, it was subzero outside. We lived approximately ten miles from the ballroom. After my wife wrangled my two little ones into their dress clothes and tried valiantly to place them in their car seats, she started the ignition on the car. *Rut rut rut! Rut rut rut!* Wouldn't you know it? The darn car wouldn't start on this arctic day. After some due diligence, my wife was able to get the car started. Onward to the event they would go, only to be stopped on Lake Shore Drive by a three car pile-up. Well, the momentum of the continuous stop and go of the car lulled my daughter to sleep. My boy, however, was a different story. My wife heard some retching in the backseat and, after a few minutes...*rallllphhhh*! My son threw up all over his dress clothes and into the car seat! Of course, they got there just in the nick of time, but my biggest regret was the comment that came out of me next. "Where have *you been*? It's *about* to *start*!" I do believe at the end of the celebration, my wife handed me the two kids and said, "Here y'are! I'm *done*!" Rightfully so. I would've done the same.

This story is not to discourage; it is simply to provide awareness of what our significant others go through on a daily basis so our illustrious career in the fire service can go on without a hitch. The main take-away is that the family *always* sacrifices for us. On CFD, we pick our vacation time in late Fall. This goes into effect the next calendar year. After we receive our days off, they are set in stone unless we do one of two things: we get promoted or we put in for a transfer. Ironically enough, after planning a get away with the family, there will be a transfer order or a promotion around the same time. So, the trip to the Keys that you were planning is essentially ruined. Hope you had travel insurance!

The reality of the situation is that a spouse is on their own for a 24 hour period. It is Murphy's Law that allows something to go awry at home while we are on shift. This includes, but is not limited to: sick/injured children, emergency house repairs, large financial decisions (which require both parties' input), large-scale emotional turmoil, and much *much* more. It is these times that test the relationship. The integrity of both parties will be put through the ringer. I assure you, this knowledge is not privy to the possible suitor during courtship. If it was, there would be a copious amount of dust from the person running the other way. But what is one to do if there is a dire emergency at the homestead that requires my immediate presence? The fire department preaches family first, but when stuff hits the fan, they are certainly not going to let someone go on shift. My realistic answer is, it is easier to ask for forgiveness than it is for permission. We work to live, not the other way around. This is important. Especially for those that have the firefighting gene deeply embedded in our persona; being with your family is more important. I'll say that again, *the most important thing is your family*…not the other way around.

After 20 years of service, my wife and I have established a wonderful life for our family. But being that both of us work such odd shifts, we find that leisure time gets pushed by the wayside. This is a common occurrence. It is vital to provide a well-rounded view of the world for our family. When my children were younger, it was weekly trips to the zoo. I knew every playground within a 200 mile radius. Playdates, ice skating, trips to the beach, all of these components are essential to the shaping of our children and families. But it is easy to lose track of these things. Now it is even more pertinent to make sure your kids are stimulated. With iPads and social media on the rise, it is *essential* to get some offline time. This could be found in many different ways. Weekly game nights are always a hit, or a seasonal favorite is taking our Labrador retriever to the woods and walking around. The world is your oyster.

There are times when firefighters become so wrapped up in the job that work becomes the center focus of their life. Due to the extreme nature of our profession, there is no lack of stories to go around. A common mistake, especially for new couples, is eating up precious time while talking about the job. Even though the spouse may be truly interested in these stories, it makes it hard to be present in your daily life. Being present means living for today. Enjoying the world around you as you navigate your life together. This could be planning events to do that day (like picking out home decor), or going out to dinner and discussing life's wonders. A common mistake that firefighters do is discuss the fire service component of their life throughout most of their day. To them, they are excited about their profession. But to others, the conversation may become tedious and repetitive. In practice, I have found that devoting (at most) an hour or less to talking about the fire service will allow us to be present with each other. Getting fire talk out of the way will make way for new experiences. I have found that this is a great practice with couples who focus on their careers more than anything else. Earmarking time to discuss the happenings at work will leave room for a plethora of other conversations.

Family functions are usually a bone of contention within fire service families. Actually, any gathering that involves having the family attend something, whether it be a holiday party, church, a wedding, etc. usually creates turmoil due to some folks misunderstanding the absence of a family member. More often than not, a firefighter will miss a family function due to being on shift. Our shifts on CFD are 24 hours on duty (that's 7 AM to 7 AM the next day) and 48 hours off duty. So, one whole day and night followed by two whole days off. This is called the Three Platoon System. Inevitably, there will be holidays where the firefighter will be on shift. This means that the spouse must dress the children, shuttle them to the party, and explain to the family why *you* are not in attendance. It doesn't always go well, and the spouse is left holding the answers and the guilt.

One of the most common emotions that people come to my office with is *anger*. They will say that they don't know why, but they have felt very angry recently. It is important to note that anger is a secondary emotion. This does not mean that it is any less important; it simply means that there are other things that are causing the anger. The primary emotion is fear, so in session we will process what they may be afraid of in hopes that this will resolve the anger. The Gottman Institute illustrates this by describing the Anger Iceberg. When you look at an iceberg, it is normal to see a small amount of ice jutting through the surface of the water. A careful eye will see that *most* of the iceberg is submerged underneath the water. The anger someone may feel is really only on the surface, while below there can be a multitude of problems that are exacerbating it. The key to this is to find the reason why someone is feeling angry and correct *that*, rather than trying to deal with the anger itself.

This becomes hindersome when a firefighter has children. Those that have them know that raising a child, much less raising multiple children, is a feat unto itself. In the beginning, there are sleepless nights as the child is still feeding throughout the night. When the child gets older, they are continuously pushing boundaries. This can be tedious in nature, as it involves disciplining the child. When a child acts out, there is nothing more frustrating than them not listening to you. The conundrum lies with a rain or shine methodology. Firefighters are either home quite a lot, or they are on shift. It comes to being away from home a third of the year. It is easy for children to play favorites as they navigate the discipline process. They can play favorites with their parents, favoring one over the other, or they can play them against each other ("Mom said I can go to the concert," when clearly she has *not* allowed this).

And, of course, there are missed holiday concerts, plays, and recitals. It sometimes takes an act of congress for a firefighter to take time off from work, so it is easier (and commonplace) for them to just miss events. This becomes hard for not only the child, but for the parent. Who wouldn't want to see their child perform as the second hyena in the 4th grade presentation of "The Lion King" (Allers, 1994)? In addition to this, the burden falls on the spouse. They must get them ready and prepared for the show and explain that, again, Mommy or Daddy will not be there. This absenteeism is a common occurrence in the world of the firefighter.

I have been lucky. My wife has permitted me to come home and sleep after my shift. Not everyone is lucky enough to have this luxury. Some people have side jobs that they go to immediately after their shift. Others have young children that they must attend to. For most of my career, I have worked in very busy firehouses. A shift in the city may include responding to anywhere in the ballpark of 10-20 calls in a 24 hour period. Many of these calls may be after midnight. When I get home from shift, my wife will always ask me the obligatory question, "How was your night?" This is code for, "How many calls did you do after midnight?" This is vital information for her so she knows if she is on her own for just the morning or into the afternoon. You see, firehouse sleep is not quality sleep. When we enter the firehouse in the morning to report to shift, our pulse and blood pressure goes up. This is our sympathetic nervous system doing its job to ensure that we are game ready throughout our tour of duty. When nighttime comes, depending on the house, there might be multiple rigs. Even if your rig does not turn a wheel, there may be others that are in your house that get toned out. For those that have never experienced this, I will describe it. Have you ever been asleep at home, quietly in your bed, when you are woken up by your significant other because your alarm clock has not gone off and you are now late to work? The immediate fear that sets in as you jump out of bed and run to splash water on your face is the *exact* feeling when the tones go off for a fire at 2:30 in the morning. So, my after shift naps allow me to recharge and ultimately be a better person the next day when I am with my family. The take home is that not everyone is awarded this opportunity. The outcome can be detrimental as they navigate their day being tired and exhausted while making decisions at their home or side job.

Marriage in itself is challenging. Being married to a firefighter can provide obstacles that are not necessarily found within a marriage to a nine to fiver. When I was dating my wife, we took a trip to New York to pay our respects at the sacred Ground Zero where the events unfolded on that catastrophic day in September. The pile of twisted metal and ruins was excavated and all that remained was hallowed ground that was still raw like an open wound. I was in uniform, so they allowed me to walk down to the location. She turned to me, pontificating about what those brave firefighters did on that fateful morning and asked me if I would risk *my* life if put in a position to do so at work. Without hesitation, I told her, "It's what I signed up for." Like a regal queen seeing her king go off to defend the kingdom, she replied, "Thank you, I *just* wanted to hear you say it; now I know." Being the spouse of someone that goes to work and may not return has to be the most wretched, anxiety-riddled feeling imaginable. Throughout my career, my wife has told me she knew what she would say at my funeral. It was a story. When I first got to the West Side as a firefighter, I went to a fire. I was assigned to the hydrant. Fire was blowing out the kitchen window. We arrived on scene, and I grabbed my tools and made the hydrant. I grabbed my air pack, knelt by the front door, put my facemask and helmet on, and like a lightning bolt, followed the line into the fire. Apparently, I followed the line too far and was on top of the other firefighters who were successfully darkening down the fire. I heard, "Gregg? Is that *you*?" from my fellow comrades. Of course, we could not see our hands in front of our faces due to the smoke conditions (unfortunately, Hollywood would have you believe otherwise). "Yup! It's me! What can I do?" I responded. "Can you back up a couple feet? You're on my *back*!" he shouted. My wife loved this story and was prepared to share it upon my demise. Maybe it was her way of coming to terms with my potential death and putting a humorous spin to it, but this is what goes through someone's head when they are married to a firefighter.

My firefighter couples are near and dear to me. I try to instill insight to them as a firefighter, as a counselor, and as a spouse. I believe they listen because I am living the same life they are. Of course, we do not live in a vacuum; every marriage is unique. One allegory I like to use to illustrate a key component to a successful marriage is the two vessels. There are times in your spouse's life where they will not be their best, and there will be times when you are not on your A-game. It is up to one of you to make sure to be the strong one. It is like two vessels that are filled with water. Sometimes, both of your vessels will be full. Enjoy these times. But more often than not, one of your vessels will be depleted and the other's will be full. It is during these times that you must pour your water into your spouse's vessel to make sure they are able to survive. Surely it will be reciprocated at a later date in life.

Many families consider their pet as part of the family. This is certainly true in my house. My children grew up with Billy. Billy was a 90 pound black Labrador who was as loyal as he was obedient. Nothing, however, could help his addiction to playing catch with a tennis ball. He became a part of the family, gracing holiday cards and coming with us to social gatherings. He was a fixture in our lives for 15 years. Even though we had to say goodbye to him, he was a joy to have. Billy taught us about unconditional love. There was nothing better than coming home from shift and seeing him waiting by the back door, wagging. Although he knew I was tired, he would play bow into downward dog. I would scratch his ears. This little exchange when I got home would prove to be cathartic for me. With the chaos left behind from my shift, Billy would be my welcome back to reality. He was the corridor for my mental shift from firefighter to father. So, then it was shower, send the kids to the bus, and then retreat to my bed. Billy would sleep lengthwise against my body as I would nod off.

Although my wife would tell you she enjoys it when I'm on shift because she gets a night of rest (I am like a salmon swimming upstream in my sleep...and I also talk), I feel her time with Billy in my absence was cathartic for her as well. After 17 years of marriage, I have found that when my wife is gone for a conference out of state, the bed is lonely. Her presence is there, but she is not. When I look over to her side of the bed in her absence, I feel as though I am walking without my wallet. I know I'm supposed to have it, but when I reach down into my pocket, it is not there. That feeling sucks. I would think that even though she likes to pretend that it's a good thing when I am on shift, the absence is loud like a screaming mouse.

When Billy passed away, it was harder than I expected. There was a lot of ugly crying going on in the Bagdade household. After we picked up the pieces of our grief, we found someone that bred Labradors. I came back from a fishing trip with my father to meet the dog who would fill the big paws of my beloved Billy. My wife wanted to name the little mousy guy with Dumbo ears Stanley (partly because we liked the name, but mostly because we are hockey fans. Go Blackhawks!), but my daughter wanted nothing to do with that nonsense. "So, what do *you* want to name him?" we asked accusatorily. She decided on Apollo, firstly for its reference to the Greek Mythological hero, and secondly, as a nod to the space program for which she had an affinity.

Apollo grew up to be rambunctious, loyal, and quite the cuddler, much like his predecessor. But, regardless of his 80 pound stature, he considers himself a lap dog, lying across our lap and making sure to touch all of those around him in one fell swoop; he loves the attention. With the introduction of a newly emerging pandemic in 2020, my family (like many others across the world) suffered severely to keep their mental health in check. COVID-19, as it would be known, robbed my children of certain benchmarks for their childhood: graduation from 8th Grade, a trip to Washington DC, the school play. Days were spent on the computer attending class via Zoom sessions. This occurring all when the intellectuals were telling us to limit screen time on electronics. Apollo provided his due diligence to ensure that my children were loved and cared for. He was there for them in between their classes. They would sit at their desks all day, staring at a computer screen and listening to a teacher that was broadcasting class for 30 other students. Apollo was always there, sitting on the couch waiting for them to wrap their tired, frustrated arms around his scruff. He provided unlimited licks and they *loved* his moans in approval.

There is a bonafide reason why there are emotional support animals. They provide unconditional love to those that need it. That, in itself, is reason enough to get a comfort animal. It matters not what type of animal brings you joy, feather or fur, skin or scales, having one is an asset to anyone's mental health. They are often used for anxiety, panic attacks, PTSD, as well as social phobias. It is not required for someone to register their animal in order to yield all the benefits they have for us. It is well known that dogs reduce stress, anxiety and depression, will help with loneliness, and encourage you to exercise (National Alliance on Mental Health, 2021). The benefits of having someone in the house that depends on you are astronomical.

On my days off, I like to take Apollo to a 12-acre, dog friendly forest preserve. It is super hard to find greenspace within the city for a dog to run around, so traveling to dog friendly areas is essential. Ever since my children were young, we found going to this dog park was a great affair. The only essentials: a ball, a towel, and a dog. The dog friendly area is chock full of land for us to navigate. There are trails, ponds, and fields. It's like an amusement park for dogs! Getting out, walking the trails and seeing how happy Apollo is brings a smile to my face every time.

As we work our fire department jobs, we can get caught up in a tumultuous web of work. Much like our sisters and brothers in blue (that's Police Officers for you playing at home), it is hard to turn off being a firefighter. When we are out to dinner at a restaurant and someone collapses, it is inevitably an off duty firefighter who will step up to render care to the victim. It is quite hard to turn it off. When my wife and I go on vacation, we play a little game. We make up what our jobs are (she is a nurse, by the way), so as not to draw attention to the call gods who might be wanting us to spring into action on our booze cruise in St. Lucia. Our favorite faux occupation is dolphin trainers at SeaWorld. Hopefully we will never be called out to rescue a sea lion under our thinly veiled white lie! Having a pet can allow us to unwind from the rigors of shift in a healthy manner. Caring for these loving animals will allow you to nurture while getting nurtured yourself.

SO, WHAT DO I DO NOW?

"There are places I'll remember all my life though some have changed. Some forever, not for better, some have gone and some remain."

(Lennon/McCartney, 1965)

When I first got on the job, I was told by an old-time firefighter, "Hang on tight, kid. It goes by quick!" With the blink of an eye, I am trying to make my next moves away from the fire department. I cannot begin to tell you how quickly time has flown. I look back at the last 20 years and it was as if I went to bed as a candidate and woke up ready for retirement. I think routine plays a big hand in this. As you know, the fire service is paramilitary in nature.

0700-0800 hrs – Check out my air pack and my equipment

0800 hrs – Roll call

0815-0900 hrs – Housework

0900-1100 hrs – Daily rig responsibilities (clean ladders, wax rig)

1200 hrs – Lunch

Lunch. Everyone loves lunch. It is the first break in the day that allows a communal feast with all the fixings of a cohesive family (or dysfunctional, depending how you look at it). Most firehouses eat family style. You get your plate. You get your own food. You clean your plate. You clean the kitchen. The process is much like a ballet. "What do you want me to do?" is not asked. It is more like finding what is not done and doing it. If someone is on the dishes, you mop. If someone is mopping, you put leftovers away. If the leftovers are being put away, you try to steal the mop away from the person mopping (but a good firefighter *never* gives up their tools, so they will surely not give up their mop). Mixed in during all this, there is banter like no other. Conservatives and liberals discussing how the other is simply nuts. A guy is building a deck at home and one guy is arguing that the posts need to be dug four feet while another guy is sure that it should be four and a half feet because he dug them four feet before and it wasn't enough. Two others are mad at the first shift for sticking them with filling up the fuel tank. I know it sounds exhausting. But to firefighters, the firehouse banter is an essential part of the day.

Lately, we have had ride-alongs from the academy stopping by. A ride along is when a candidate will ride with a rig for an undisclosed amount of time to get a taste of what the job is like away from the textbooks or drill hall. I'd have to say that the best experiences for these individuals is two-fold: 1) When at the firehouse, the personalities of everyone are chock-full of character and zest, 2) When we are on a call, everyone becomes another person. Professional, precise, and perfect. As soon as the call is over, we can all return to the typical doofuses we were prior. Sometimes I am in awe of the men and women that I work with. They are matriarchs and patriarchs of their own family: coaching baseball in the summer or making sure their household is neat, fed, and in control. Others have their own businesses: general contractors, teaching classes to mold young minds, owners of restaurants and bars. The list goes on. On CFD, there is a conglomerate of races and ethnicities that create such a rich environment even NATO could learn a thing or two about getting along with someone who may look at the number 6 and think it's a 9. That's called perspective. Race, religion, gender, sexual orientation, these things matters not. When it's time to go to work, everyone simply gets it done.

When someone is new to the job, they may place a fire department sticker on their vehicle or they may wear a blue t-shirt that represents their firehouse. This is considered company pride. "Yup! I *am* a paramedic at Ambulance 10, out of Engine 95's house…Busiest ambo in the nation!" After all, who wouldn't be proud of their job if it involved saving lives? So, the tryst continues. You go on vacation with your family in Cancun. Don't forget to pack those fire department t-shirts. Gotta represent the old CFD when I'm on the beach. Eventually, days off are spent with guys and gals from the firehouse: lunch at the local watering hole, nights down to the casino, and weekend trips with your families to the water slide park. It becomes too hard to explain what it actually is that you do to your high school friends, so those visits become obsolete. This leaves room to spend more time with people that get you. They understand what it is to be up all night doing call after call on New Year's Eve. They get that you won't be showing up to Christmas dinner because you are on shift, and they won't make a big deal about it. They will take you to the bars without asking a gosh forsaken thing about your failed marriage, your rising debt, your ill son, all because you are part of a brotherhood and sisterhood that others do not understand. And once you're in, you're in for life!

Being a firefighter is a culture that is ingrained in us from the beginning. It carries on in us throughout our career. It almost becomes our identity. "Who's coming with us to dinner?" a friend might ask. "Oh, it's Gregg, the firefighter." Rarely will people say "Tim, the Financial Advisor," or "Jack, the Attorney." We wear this hat and we wear it proudly. This identity may also be a cross that we all must bear. To put it fatalistically, when we retire, what do we have to show for ourselves minus the years in the fire service? When I got on the job in 2001, you couldn't pry people from the job if you tried. People were not leaving to retire. In Chicago, we can actually begin receiving a portion of our pension after the age of 50 and having 20 years of service. Ultimately, it is mandatory to retire at the age of 63. So, somewhere in between we have the opportunity to collect a modest pension and enjoy life, right?

The generation of firefighters that came before us would not hear of this. We would ask, "Why don't you just take your pension and retire?" The question would come up regularly. "And do what?? This is the *best* job in the *world*!" or the more disturbing answer, "I'd have to spend more time with my wife! We don't want *that*!" the seasoned firefighter would respond, feeling satisfied. That would just lead to more questions. I don't know what is more disturbing: not wanting to enjoy retirement after you have put well earned time into the pension, or refusing to spend it with your spouse after they have endured your working conditions after all these years? Both are troubling to me.

The long and the short of the situation is, even when we are afforded the opportunity to retire, we don't want to take it. But here is a notion that scares me: Are those that *do* retire prepared to live a life of normalcy away from the fire service? You see, being in the fire service for a whole career is not unlike being in the military, or being institutionalized for that matter. There are known issues that arise in both of these conditions that lend themselves to needing outside help. No wonder the rate of suicide for retired firefighters is sky high. For some time I thought about teaching a class to those that were ready for retirement. I felt it necessary to prevent the amount of retirees that might flounder when they get to that age. Showing them that a little preparation can go a long way might help someone redirect their future and prevent them from going down a lonely road. When a firefighter retires, they will (more often than not) revisit their old firehouse to see how things are going. This is not uncommon and is understandable considering the circumstances. After a while, they will continue to show up, and as the shift may change through promotions and transfers, try to relive the good old days. I would affectionately refer to these guys as Back-Door Retirees, because they would enter the firehouse through the back door. There are multitudes of them in existence who simply cannot move forward and who relive the past as much as they can. What has happened to them is they were part of the fire service and now they are not.

Ultimately, there needs to be some sort of acclimation process that will show these future retirees that there are things they can do in order to get on with their lives. Because of the ability to retire in their 50s, these individuals can be relatively young. Even for those that go to the very end and retire at the mandatory age, 63 is hardly old. There are plenty of activities that they can do in order to stay active. For example, there is an organization that caters to retirees and helps them get involved in emergency preparedness. An example of this is CERT, or Community Emergency Response Team. They are the boots on the ground for natural disasters and are trained in "basic disaster response such as fire safety, light search and rescue, team organization, and disaster medical operations" (Hopkins Minnesota, 2022). Most retired firefighters would shine in a role like this, due to their decade spanning career in emergency services. They meet regularly in order to keep up with their training, and there is a social interaction component as well.

Another option for them could be learning an instrument. There is a growing community of fire service bagpipe bands who play for such events as St. Patrick's Day, benefits, retirement parties, and more. A brief history of bagpipes in the fire service explains that when immigrants came over to the United States, it was the Irish and Scottish who took the most dangerous jobs. Many of them became police officers and firefighters. With them, they brought their instruments and so, to honor this tradition, bagpipe bands have become commonplace within the fire service community. The nice thing about bagpipe bands is they meet weekly and keep the mind sharp by learning how to read music and play either the Great Highland Bagpipes or several different types of drums. This could keep a retiree busy for many years to come.

Realistically speaking, there are a multitude of jobs that a retiree could do. From emergency room technician to local government positions; the sky's the limit. More importantly, the retiree will keep sharp and have a purpose in life. One issue that people have when they retire is they do not prepare for the time off. When someone retires, they are very young. 50-63 years old is young. There are still many years of life in those old bones. More importantly, if the person is not occupied with a task, they will find themselves in disrepair, asking "What is my purpose in life?" or "What can I do to fill my day?" Some retirees end up traveling. This is a wonderful way to see new cultures and spend time in exotic places. However, traveling may become costly, and there is still the question of what to do when you get back from a trip.

I was at the firehouse one time and a back-door retiree came in to have lunch. We all asked how he was doing. (He had retired roughly one year before). "I'm fine...*now!*" was his reply. He spoke about not having anything prepared when he retired. Months were spent at the bar, drinking and finding social events. After that, he started watching Netflix. Days upon days of binge watching shows. When he became wary of this, he began showing up at firehouses looking for companionship and something to fill up his day. Finally, he visited old family and friends. After he wore out his welcome, he realized that he needed something to do. He was 55 years old and only knew the education that the fire service had provided for him. After much thinking, he decided to enroll in a program that teaches heating, ventilation, and air conditioning (HVAC) installation and repair. He *loves* it! It keeps him busy and out of trouble.

Because of its paramilitary nature, many social programs regarding mental health are cleaved from the four major military services and adapted for the fire service. For example, peer support programs and PTSD awareness and treatment have their roots in the military. Information has recently been shared regarding these issues and has spilled over, benefitting our firefighters. One such program I'd like to see adapted is the reintegration of military personnel into society after spending time in combat. These programs traditionally involve social support, work programs, and counseling. Ideally, if this was to become portable for the fire service, it would have to be scaled down. This could be done in an eight hour class prior to retirement. It could be mandatory for all retirees to take this class. Making them aware of the pitfalls that lie ahead of them could benefit these retirees for years to come. There could be discussion about finding age appropriate tasks that satisfy their physical, mental, and social domains. Finally, local organizations could be present to recruit individuals that are interested in this vision. The goal is to set the retiree up for success and steer them in the right direction rather than them going down a road of despair.

BE LIKE GEORGE

"And in the end, the love you take is equal to the love you make."
(Lennon & McCartney, 1969)

The mind of a firefighter is quite the anomaly. While they continuously do heroic acts, the chorus will adamantly oppose this, singing the song of the humble man. Even in everyday practice, they are the ones who will come over and repair your hot water heater when it goes on the fritz. They are the coaches of your kids' softball team. They provide the jumper cables to your broken down car and give you a jump. There is no lesson plan that dictates this in the fire academy; they simply do this without pause. It is innate. Like a mother's instinct to check on her newborn overnight. Throughout literature, there is a notion that is referred to as an archetype. *The Oxford Dictionary* (Oxford University Press, n.d.) refers to this as, "a very typical example of a certain person or thing." Well, I feel that the firefighter should be represented as what is called the Everyman (Everywoman) archetype. The Everyman is the person next door, the working stiff, the regular person. They embody empathy, humbleness, and a lack of pretense. Think of the characters that Bill Murray tends to play in such movies as *Stripes* or *Ghostbusters*. He is like you and me. When you watch these films, there is no large jump from assuming that our own selves could be placed in this very position. But the Everyman Archetype that really resonates with the firefighter is that of Jimmy Stewart in the holiday favorite, *It's A Wonderful Life* (Capra,1946).

The story takes us through the life of George Bailey. His life is riddled with problems which bring him to a bridge where he contemplates suicide. At this very moment, a car falls off the bridge and crashes in the icy water below. George dives in after and pulls out Clarence, who happens to be his guardian angel. Clarence shows George what life would be like if he was not around. George sees the bedlam of this alternate universe and decides to choose life. George is the Everyman in this holiday favorite, the anti-hero. For it is *he* that struggles with the toils of everyday life. It is *he* that tries to keep it together as his business is faltering. It is *he* that must manage his work life as well as his family life while he is mentally struggling. He is just like the firefighter...the Everyman.

With the determination to get the job done, it is the firefighter that will do so. When they arrive on the scene and check the hydrant with their tools in the driving snow, it may be frozen. It is their perseverance that will run to the next hydrant and drag even more hose to make sure their brothers and sisters on the inside of the house fire get their water. They will then run to the rig, put on their air pack and follow the line in to relieve their comrade on the pipe. Spent from this gargantuan feat, they will continue to serve their community for the rest of their shift.

Throughout this book, I sincerely hope that my voice was heard. For it is the loudest chick in the nest that wins the worm from their mother. I must reiterate and highlight the important factors that I wish to bestow on you, the reader. Firefighters see bad stuff. When someone says that this is what they signed up for, there is certainly much truth to this. However, most people will only see a few traumatic events in their lifetime. A firefighter may see hundreds in their career. Physiologically, their brains will file these events under corrupt files and force the individual to deal with the repercussions in their own rite. When the resources simply are not there for them to appropriately cope with the very bad stuff, they are forced to commence coping in a maladaptive way. Drinking, drugs, unsafe sexual exploits, and excessive gambling are all ways that firefighters cope with their newfound trauma because it is convenient. It is available. It is what they know. Their relationships with others, including spouses, friends, and family, will certainly be affected, and they will be forced to navigate the outcome on their own. Much of this turmoil will be enhanced by a stigma perpetuated by a hundred plus years of machismo, competition, and accepting things the way they have always been. It does not have to be this way anymore.

When time passes, so do accomplishments, accolades, and other things of that sort. I will not be the first, nor will I be the last, to support change within the fire service. But the time has arrived. Professional journals, trade magazines, and the like are promoting mental health for our firefighters every chance they can get. Even at the firehouse kitchen table, where all the worlds' problems are solved, firefighters are acknowledging that there are other ways to cope with their job-related ills. The fire service is changing. I recall coming up, learning the job, taking classes, and finding busy spots so I could get real on-the-job training. It was really a baptism by fire. But we can learn from these new recruits, for they are much more in-tune with their mental wellbeing. They know that it is just as important to keep in touch with their therapist regularly as it is to receive an annual physical. Going to a counselor should not occur when stuff has hit the fan. Regular counseling relieves the pressure build-up. It is a person that you can go to that is on the outside looking in. They are not emotionally invested in your issues, so they can come up with solutions that are tailor-made for you. This will benefit not only you, but the social relationships you create. For example, by having a dog that loves you unconditionally, you may find yourself growing as a human because this animal will give you unconditional love. Or you may find that at the end of your career, you will not sit on an island sipping piña coladas because you do not want to do a thing after you retire. You will become productive and join your local Lions Club, or join the CERT team, or learn to play an instrument. We can retire between the ages of 50 and 63. This is young! Very young. Certainly young enough for us to keep moving and have a sharp mind. Ultimately, the choice is yours, but the suicide rate of retirees will tell you a different story.

My three voices have spoken throughout this book. They are: my personal voice, my firefighter voice, and my counselor voice. It was my goal to intertwine the three of them to allow you to see my perspective from three angles. In counseling, we learn that there is something called parts work. I often go over this quite extensively with my clients. The person you are at the firehouse certainly isn't who you are with your spouse and children. Who you are with your friends does not correlate with who you are to your parents. The purpose of my three voices was to bestow my knowledge by revealing to you, the reader, the parts that make up me. Each part summates a whole. Sometimes, I needed to give information that a firefighter would reveal. Other times, it was me or my counselor self. It all comes to a head when push comes to shove. It is up to you to tie it all together in your mind and create a change for yourself. It is no longer helpless for us. There are avenues we can take. With this book to guide you, I assure you you will make it, even if you have a mental health mayday, from recruit through retirement.

REFERENCES

Allers, R.(Director).(1994). *The Lion King* [Film]. United States: Buena Vista Pictures.

American Psychological Association. (2020). *Publication Manual of the American Psychological Association* (7th ed.). https://doi. org/10.1037/0000165-000

Bacal, J., DePatie,D.H., Loesch, M. Griffin, T., Gunther, L. (Executive Producers).(1983-1986). *G.I. joe: A Real American Hero.* [TV series]. Sunbow Productions, Marvel Productions.

Capra, F. (Director) (1946). *It's a Wonderful Life.* [Film]. RKO Radio Pictures.

Hopkins Minnesota. (2022). *CERT: Community Emergency Response Team.* https://www.hopkinsmn.com/253/CERT-Community-Emergency-Response-Team.

Cramer, P. (2000). Defense mechanisms in psychology today: Further processes for adaptation.

American psychologist, 55(6), 637.

Hoban, R. (2021, May 4). Similar bills to help first responders with health issues are in front of legislators. They're likely to have different outcomes. *NC Health News,* https://www. northcarolinahealthnews.org

Gandhi, M. (1999). *The Collected Works of Mahatma Gandhi,* [eBook edition]. Publications Division Government of India. vol. http://www.gandhiashramsevagram.org/gandhi-literature/collected-works-of-mahatma-gandhi-volume-1-to-98.php

Gelbart, L. (Executive Producer). (1972-1983). *M*A*S*H** [TV series]. 20th Century Fox   Television.

Goldberg, A.F., et al. (Executive Producers) (2013-Present). *The Goldbergs.* [TV series]. Happy   Madison   Productions,   Sony   Pictures Television.

Harrison, G. (1968). *While my Guitar Gently Weeps.* [Album]. Apple.

Illinois Firefighter Peer Support. (2021, November 21) *Peer Support Curriculum.* http://www.iffps.org.

Lazarus, R. S., & Folkman, S. (1984). *Stress, Appraisal, and Coping.* Springer publishing company.

Lennon J. & McCartney P., (1965). *You've Got to Hide your Love Away.* [Album].Parlophone.

Lennon J. & McCartney P.,(1965). *Help!.* [Album]. Parlophone.

Lennon J. & McCartney P.,(1965). *In my Life.* [Album]. Parlophone.

Lennon J. & McCartney P.,(1967). *I am the Walrus.* [Album].Parlophone.

Lennon J. & McCartney P.,(1967). *With a Little Help from my Friends.* [Album].Parlophone.

Lennon J. & McCartney P.,(1967). *Penny Lane.* [Album].Parlophone.

Lennon J. & McCartney P.,(1967). *A Day in the Life.* [Album].Parlophone.

Lennon J. & McCartney P.,(1967). *Getting Better.* [Album]. Parlophone.

Lennon J. & McCartney P.,(1967). *Fixing a Hole.* [Album]. Parlophone.

Lennon J. & McCartney P.,(1969). *Carry that Weight.* [Album].Apple.

Lennon J. & McCartney P.,(1969). *The End.* [Album]. Apple.

Lennon J. & McCartney P.,(1970). *Let it Be.* [Album]. Apple.

Lucas, G. (Director) (1977). *Star Wars.* [Film]. Disney.

Maté, G. (2018). *In the Realm of Hungry Ghosts: Close Encounters with Addiction.* Vermilion.

Mitchell, J. T., & Everly, G. S. (1997). Critical incident stress debriefing (CISD). An Operations Manual for the Prevention of Traumatic Stress Among Emergency Service and Disaster Workers. Second Edition, Revised. Ellicott City: Chevron Publishing Corporation.

National Alliance on Mental Illness. (2021, November 21). The Power of Pet Therapy. https://nami.org/Home.

Oxford University Press. (n.d.). Everyman. In *Oxford English Dictionary.* Retrieved November 21, 2021, from https://www.oed.com.

Rankin/Bass Animated Entertainment. (Executive Producer). (1985-1988). *Thundercats.* [TV series].Lorimar Productions, Warner Bros.

Rosner, R. (Executive Producer). (1977-1983). *CHiPs* [TV series]. MGM Television.

Schaffner, F.J. (Director). (1970). *Patton* [Film]. 20th Century Fox.

Scorcese. M. (Director). (1999). *Bringing out the Dead* [Film]. Paramount Pictures.

Shapiro, F. & Forrest, M. (1997). *EMDR The Breakthrough Therapy for Overcoming Anxiety, Stress and Trauma.* New York: Basic Books

Shaw, G.B. (1962). *Androcles and the L ion.* Penguin Books.

Taylor, S. G., Katherine Renpenning, M., & Renpenning, K. M. (2011). *Self-care science, Nursing Theory and Evidence-Based Practice.* Springer Publishing Company.

van der Kolk, B. A. (2014). *The Body Keeps the Score: Brain, Mind, and Body in the Healing of Trauma.* Viking.

Wachowski, La., Wachowski, Li. (Directors). (1999) *The Matrix* [Film]. Warner Bros.

Webb, J.,Cinader, R.A., Shearer, H.L.(Executive Producers). (1972-1977). *Emergency!* [TV series]. Mark VII Limited, Universal Television

Williams, G.(2014,October 20) Stop it, I can't.[Video] Youtube. https://www.youtube.com/watch?v=57vFum4yUcE

SELECTED
MSI PRESS PUBLICATIONS

A Woman's Guide to Self-Nurturing (Romer)

Anger Anonymous (Ortman)

Anxiety Anonymous (Ortman)

Creative Aging (Vassiliadis & Romer)

Damascus amid the War (Imady)

Depression Anonymous (Ortman)

Diary of an RVer during Quarantine (MacDonald)

Divorced! (Romer)

El Poder de lo Transpersonal (Ustman)

Exercising in a Pandemic (Young)

Forget the Goal, the Journey Counts (Stites)

From Deep Within (Lewis)

Girl, You Got This! (Renz)

Harnessing the Power of Grief (Potter)

Helping the Disabled Veteran (Romer)

He's a Porn Addict...Now What? (Overbay and Shea)

How My Cat Made Me a Better Man (Feig)

How to Be a Good Mommy When You're Sick (Graves)

How to Improve Your Foreign Language Immediately (Shekhtman)

How to Live from Your Heart (Hucknall)

How to Stay Calm in Chaos (Gentile)

Lamentations of the Heart (Wells-Smith)

Life after Losing a Child (Young)

Life, Liberty, and Covid-19 (Ortman)

Living Well with Chronic Illness (Charnas)

Noah's New Puppy [K-9] (Rice, Rice, & Henderson)

Old and on Hold (Cooper)

One Simple Text… (Shaw & Brown)

Passing On (Romer)

Puertas a la Eternidad (Ustman)

Rainstorm of Tomorrow (Dong)

Recovering from Domestic Violence, Abuse, & Stalking (Romer)

Road Map to Power (Husain & Husain)

RV Oopsies (MacDonald)

Soccer Is Fun without Parents (Jonas)

Spunky Grandmas and Other Amusing Characters (Mogren)

Staying Safe While Sheltering in Place (Schnuelle, Adams, & Henderson)

Survival of the Caregiver (Snyder)

The Musings of a Carolina Yankee (Amidon)

The Pandemic and Hope (Ortman)

The Widower's Guide to a New Life (Romer)

Typhoon Honey (Girrell & Sjogren)

Widow (Romer)